Atlas of Two-Dimensional Echocardiography in Congenital Cardiac Defects

Atlas of Two-Dimensional Echocardiography in Congenital Cardiac Defects

by

G.J. VAN MILL, A.J. MOULAERT, E. HARINCK

Wilhelmina Children's Hospital
University of Utrecht
Utrecht

Illustrations by

J.W. WETSELAAR

1983 **MARTINUS NIJHOFF PUBLISHERS**
a member of the KLUWER ACADEMIC PUBLISHERS GROUP
BOSTON / THE HAGUE / DORDRECHT / LANCASTER

Distributors

for the United States and Canada: Kluwer Boston, Inc., 190 Old Derby Street, Hingham, MA 02043, USA
for all other countries: Kluwer Academic Publishers Group, Distribution Center, P.O.Box 322, 3300 AH Dordrecht, The Netherlands

Library of Congress Cataloging in Publication Data

```
Van Mill, G. J.
    Atlas of two-dimensional echocardiography in
congenital cardiac defects.

    1. Ultrasonic cardiography--Atlases.  2. Heart--
Abnormalities--Diagnosis--Atlases.  3. Pediatric
cardiology--Diagnosis--Atlases.  4. Echocardiography
--Atlases.  I. Moulaert, André J.  II. Harinck, E.
III. Title.  [DNLM: 1. Echocardiography--Atlases.
2. Heart defects, Congenital--Diagnosis--Atlases.
WG 17 M645a]
RJ423.5.U46V36  1982     618.92'12043     82-22274
```

ISBN-13: 978-94-009-6704-5   e-ISBN-13: 978-94-009-6702-1
DOI: 10.1007/978-94-009-6702-1

Copyright

FOREWORD

In a relatively short period of time two-dimensional echocardiography has become the most important non-invasive diagnostic tool in the daily practice of a pediatric cardiologist who predominantly deals with congenital structural heart disease in neonates and infants. Consequently, one-dimensional M-mode echocardiography has lost most of its importance particularly in this field. Therefore, an atlas showing exclusively two-dimensional echocardiograms of the most common and some less frequently occurring malformations appeared to be a useful addition to the existing literature. The confinement to two-dimensional imaging alone allowed an elaborate presentation of the various defects with more than 200 selected still frames and many additional explanatory drawings and diagrams. The material was collected from patients who were referred to the Department of Pediatric Cardiology of the Wilhelmina University Children's Hospital in Utrecht during a period of about 2 years. The two-dimensional echocardiographic findings were correlated with cardiac catheterization data and/or surgical procedures and/or post-mortem investigations. The necessary echocardiographic equipment was aquired with financial aid from the Dutch Heart Foundation. We are indebted to Mrs. J.W. Wetselaar for her outstanding artwork. We also thank P.D. Woltema and F.J. van Waert for the photographic reproductions, Jacomine Bosma for preparing and type-setting the entire manuscript and Dr. N. Middleton for critically reading the English text.

G.J. van Mill, M.D.
A.J. Moulaert, M.D.
E. Harinck, M.D.

CONTENTS

VIII

1. INTRODUCTION AND THE NORMAL HEART

Introduction

Echocardiography is an integral part of the non-invasive diagnosis of heart disease. In congenital structural heart disease physical examination, electrocardiography, phonocardiography and chest X-ray disclose the secondary manifestations of the disease. Real time two-dimensional echocardiography has the advantage that it can reveal the actual anatomic lesions. Therefore, it completes the non-invasive diagnosis. In skilled hands the degree of diagnostic accuracy and completeness is such that cardiac catheterizations may be postponed or even avoided in an increasing number of cases. In combination with the use of echocontrast studies in the cardiac laboratory the number and length of the angiocardiograms can be reduced.

There are a number of factors that favourably influence the application of two-dimensional echocardiography in children with cardiac disease. Firstly, the development of the modern real time echocardiographic sector scanners and, secondly, the easy access of the ultrasonic beam to the child's heart. The chest wall of infants is thin and the amount of calcium in it is small. Therefore, there is little obstruction to the ultrasound. Aerated lung tissue in front of the heart will reject the ultrasound. Fortunately, the lungs of children are normally less voluminous than those of adults so that lung tissue is confined to the side of the heart. Besides, thymus tissue, often prominent in young children, also prevents pulmonary tissue lying in front of the great arteries. Thus, for a number of reasons the ultrasonic beam can reach the heart and great arteries in children from a large precordial area known as the ultrasonic parasternal window.

When the transducer is placed on the chest wall *the ultrasonic beam is transmitted to the heart* from one confined point and is mechanically or electronically directed in such a manner that sector-like two-dimensional echocardiograms are obtained (Figure 1.1). The area in which the sector scanner can be used is not confined to the parasternal window. Other areas are the subcostal, apical and suprasternal windows (Figure 1.2). The sector scanner has given a much wider scope to the application of two-dimensional echocardiography compared with the linear array principle (1) which necessitates large transducers hardly applicable in any but the parasternal window.

For subcostal echocardiography the transducer is placed in the subxiphoid fossa or below either one of the costal arches. Hence, the ultasonic beam passes from the inferior to the superior part of the heart. This is also the case when the apical window is used in which the transducer is positioned at the apex of the heart. When the transducer is placed in the suprasternal fossa the great arteries and the pulmonary veins can be viewed from a cranial aspect. Thus, the sector scanner allows two-dimensional echocardiographic views of the heart and great vessels from several directions (2). In infants the images practically always allow accurate description of the normal and abnormal cardiac anatomy.

The apparatus used for the production of echocardiograms in this atlas was the Mark V sector scanner with 3 and 5 mHz transducers from Advanced Technology Laboratories (ATL) in Bellevue, Washington, U.S.A. The real time images are displayed on a monitor and recorded by a video system. The images can be reviewed at normal speed, in slow motion or as still frames. The examples displayed are photographs taken from selected still frames. It should be appreciated that the quality of the echocardiograms on the still frames is inferior to that of the real time imaging.

To compensate for this to some extent the echocardiograms have been extensively labelled and many explanatory drawings added.

For the nomenclature and image orientation the recommendations of the American Society of Echocardiography (3) have been adhered to as much as possible. For accurate orientation of the images there should be no ambiguity about what is left, right, superior and inferior. All the sector planes are displayed on the monitor with the narrow angle above independent of the echocardiographic window used. Therefore, the images from the subcostal and the apical windows show the heart upside down. In this atlas these images have been reversed to portray the heart in a normal upright position. In the most modern instruments the image on the monitor can be inverted or switched from left to right during the investigation. Rotation of the images through 90° would be a further improvement and should be recommended to the manufacturers.

To analyse the normal cardiac anatomy and the exact nature of the various cardiac anomalies, all the previously mentioned ultrasonic windows should be routinely used. With the multiple two-dimensional images the investigator should be able to compose a three dimensional structure.

This atlas is intended to make the reader acquainted with the various echocardiographic planes of normal and congenitally malformed hearts. Thereby, the authors have assumed that the reader is to a certain extent familiar with the normal and abnormal cardiovascular anatomy.

In the first part of this atlas several commonly used two-dimensional echocardiographic views of the normal heart are described. The next part deals with the two-dimensional echocardiograms of the most frequently occurring congenital cardiac defects. On the final pages the echocardiograms of congenital cardiac defects less frequently seen are presented without any pretence of completeness.

The normal heart

The interventricular septum is an important intracardiac structure which can be accurately visualized by two-dimensional echocardiography. Because the interventricular septum is a curved structure it is not confined to one echocardiographic plane. Hence, it should be viewed from several echocardiographic windows. To describe the interventricular septum exactly the classification of Anderson (4) is useful. In this classification the interventricular septum is divided into four integral components viz the membranous septum, inlet septum, outlet septum and the trabecular septum, whereby the last three parts constitute the muscular septum (Figure 1.3). The inlet septum is the posterior part of the interventricular septum. Because of its posterior extension it divides the inflow tracts of both ventricles. It is best visualized from the subcostal window where the ultrasonic beam strikes this part of the interventricular septum perpendicularly or almost perpendicularly. The outlet septum and the trabecular septum are situated anteriorly. These parts of the interventricular septum should be viewed from the parasternal window from where the ultrasonic beam is directed perpendicularly at those structures. The outlet septum is located directly beneath the semilunar valves and separates the outflow tracts of the ventricles. The trabecular septum is the remaining part of the muscular septum and is situated more apically. On the right side of the heart the trabecular septum is divided from the inlet septum by the trabecula septomarginalis. The three components of the muscular septum converge to the membranous septum which is located in the medial wall of the left ventricular outflow tract, directly beneath the aortic valve. On the right side of the membranous septum the septal leaflet of the tricuspid valve is attached.

The first cross-section described is the familiar long axis view of the heart. It concerns the plane of the left ventricular apex to the aorta used for many years to obtain the M-mode scans. The long axis connects the apex of the heart with the aorta in a left inferior to right superior direction. When a view that is perpendicular to the frontal plane of the patient's chest coincides with the long axis of the heart the long axis plane is visualized.

In Figure 1.4 the heart is shown in an upright position in a box representing a diagrammatic chest. The frontal plane is indicated in a smaller box by a diagrammatic torso. The small black triangle denotes the position of the transducer. The long axis plane is indicated in the diagrammatic chest. The long axis view is drawn with bold lines. This representation of the long axis view corresponds with the image orientation of the original Rotterdam linear array system, i.e. with the ascending aorta upright, the apex of the heart pointing caudally with the anterior right ventricle on the left side of the image. This is probably the most universal and logical presentation of the long axis of the heart. Unfortunately, this is not customary in two-dimensional echocardiography. In this atlas the ascending aorta is not directing superiorly but, according to the recommendations of the American Society of Echocardiography, to the right of the echocardiogram. For an anatomical appreciation of the long axis view of the heart on the echocardiogram the diagrammatic representation should be turned through 90° to the right with the ascending aorta directed to the right. Analysis of the long axis view reveals, directly beneath the transducer and underneath the chest wall, the right ventricular outflow tract which is seen in transverse cross-section. Therefore, the valves of the right heart are normally not visualized in this view. The pulmonary valve is situated slightly superior and to the left of the plane of cross-section. The tricuspid valve is positioned inferiorly and to the right of that plane. Posterior to the right ventricular outflow tract the entire left heart is seen in cross-section, displaying the left atrium behind the ascending aorta and the left ventricle with the mitral valve.

Since the long axis plane is perpendicular to the frontal plane, only the actual anterior and posterior structures are visualized, and the medial and lateral parts of the heart cannot be seen. The anterior wall of the aorta is continuous with the interventricular septum. This part of the interventricular septum, directly beneath the aortic valve, belongs to the outlet septum with the trabecular septum more apically situated.

In the dorsal region the posterior wall of the left atrium and the left ventricle is visualized. The pulmonary veins are not seen because they enter the left atrium to the right and to the left of the long axis plane. Sometimes, the right pulmonary artery may be seen just superior to the left atrium. The descending aorta may be visualized as it passes posterior to the left atrium as an oblong or round structure. The coronary sinus, transversely cut in

the atrioventricular sulcus, may also be seen in this view, particularly if it is wide (Figure 1.5). The posterior leaflet of the mitral valve, as viewed in Figure 1.4, originates at the junction of the wall of the left atrium and the left ventricle. It is inserted inferiorly into a papillary muscle. The papillary muscles are usually not seen because the long axis plane often cuts exactly between the medial and lateral papillary muscles. The anterior mitral valve leaflet is in direct continuity with the posterior wall of the aorta. Consequently, this continuity identifies that atrioventricular valve as the mitral valve. The great artery in this plane can also be identified as the aorta by its typical linear ascending course parallel to the frontal plane.

In the aortic root the aortic valve is visualized as a faint linear echo parallel to the aortic walls. This diastolic closure line should be centrally situated and represents the parts of the aortic cusps which are perpendicular to the ultrasonic beam.

Another long axis view is shown in Figure 1.6, displaying a wide ascending aorta. The transverse section of the descending aorta is clearly visualized posterior to the left atrium. The descending aorta is easily identified during the real time imaging because of its arterial pulsations and, when the transducer is shifted from the transverse to the longitudinal cross-section, by its typical descending course.

The last mentioned manipulation with the transducer provides the parasternal sagittal cross-section. This plane has a vertical direction and it is perpendicular to the frontal plane. As such the plane lies parallel and to the left of the spinal column. The posteriorly traversing main pulmonary artery and the descending aorta with its straight caudal course are simultaneously visualized (Figure 1.7). The diagrammatic chest should be turned a quarter to the right to match the exact image orientation of the corresponding echocardiogram. The long pulsating space behind the heart can easily be recognized as the descending aorta. The right ventricular outflow tract is situated directly beneath the transducer. The pulmonary valve may also be recognized in this view. The typical antero-posterior direction of the main pulmonary artery is obvious. The left atrium is situated in the small angle depicted by the main pulmonary artery and the descending aorta. The

4

apical part of the left ventricle is also visible. The subpulmonary part of the outlet septum is shown just below the pulmonary valve. More apically it is continuous with the trabecular septum. If the visual quality of this view is good a potential persistent ductus, coarctation of the aorta or subpulmonary ventricular septal defect may be recognized. If the quality of the precordial i.e. parasternal sagittal view is inadequate the subcostal window may be tried to image a similar sagittal view.

The next cross-section to be described is the long axis view of the right ventricle. To obtain this view the left ventricular long axis plane can be used as a reference point. As already mentioned this plane of cross-section is perpendicular to the frontal plane. From this position the ultrasonic beam should be directed towards the right. This visualizes the right atrium and the inflow tract of the right ventricle (Figure 1.8). For the image orientation of this cross-section the patient should be viewed from an inferior and right sided position. This view clearly shows the tricuspid valve and ring. Therefore, it should be used to observe a potential prolapse of the tricuspid valve. The anterior papillary muscle, inserted into the apex of the right ventricle, is often readily recognized in this view.

The short axis planes are perpendicular to the long axis of the heart. Hence, the transducer must be turned from the long axis view through an angle of 90° to the short axis view. Figure 1.9 demonstrates a transverse cross-section at the level of the mitral valve. The circle-like shape of the left ventricle is clearly demonstrated. The interventricular septum is convex to the right indicating a normal pressure-relationship between the two ventricles. The trabecular septum is seen anteriorly and is posteriorly continuous with the inlet septum. The demarcation between the inlet- and trabecular septum is not clearly defined echocardiographically because the trabecula septomarginalis, bordering this demarcation on the right side, normally cannot be visualized. The mitral valve is open and the two leaflets are clearly separated from each other. The typical 'fish mouth' appearance of the bicuspid atrioventricular valve marks that valve as the mitral valve. The right side of the heart is divided into right atrium and right ventricle by the

tricuspid valve. In real-time imaging the mitral valve movements can be accurately observed and abnormalities e.g. a cleft in the anterior leaflet are readily recognized or refuted. The closed mitral valve is seen in Figure 1.10a. The early opening phase of the mitral valve leaflets is seen in Figure 1.10b and in Figure 1.10c the valve is completely open. The anterior leaflet is clearly intact. At a lower level the valve leaflets are continuous via the chordae tendineae with the papillary muscles. A transverse cross-section of the two left ventricular papillary muscles is shown in Figure 1.11. The structures are referred to as the medial or right and the lateral or left papillary muscle and are unmistakably separated from each other. Both muscles are normally of equal size. The arrangement of these papillary muscles and the typical insertion into the dorsal and lateral ventricular walls clearly identify that chamber as the left ventricle. In congenital structural defects of the mitral valve both papillary muscles are inserted closer together and at a more superior level into the posterior wall of the left ventricle than in normal cases. Occasionally, the two papillary muscles have merged into one muscle bundle.

As mentioned earlier a transverse cross-section of the coronary sinus may be visualized in the atrioventricular sulcus on the long axis view. In the short axis view a wide horizontally traversing coronary sinus, longitudinally cut, can be traced towards the right atrium (Figure 1.12 and 1.13).

By shifting the transducer cranially the semilunar valves can be simultaneously visualized. The three aortic leaflets are clearly visible in the cross-section in Figure 1.14. In the closed position they display a typical 'mercedes' sign on the echocardiogram. The posterior leaflet of the pulmonary valve is situated anteriorly and to the left of the aortic valve and is simultaneously seen with the aortic leaflets. Continuous with the commissure between the right and non-coronary aortic cusps the partition between the right atrium and right ventricle i.e. the tricuspid valve is observed. The small membranous interventricular septum is situated directly beneath this commissure in the medial wall of the left ventricular outflow tract. The atrial septum is not conspicuous on the echocardiogram, therefore its normal location is indicated on the corresponding drawings. The left atrium is separated from the main pulmonary artery by the atrio-pulmonic sulcus tissue.

When the transducer is placed just above the level of the aortic valve the origin of the coronary arteries may sometimes be visualized (Figure 1.15).

Tilting the ultrasonic beam cranially the main pulmonary artery with its left and right branches may be recognized (Figure 1.16). To understand the image orientation of the echocardiographic still frame the reader should appreciate the cross-section in the diagrammatic chest as if he were looking at it from underneath. Persistent ductus arteriosus can also be looked for in this view. Normally, it is seen as a communication of the main pulmonary artery, near the origin of the left pulmonary artery, and the descending aorta which is visualized in transverse cross-section in this view.

The next cross-section to be dealt with is the four chamber view. This view visualizes simultaneously the two atria and the two ventricles. The four chamber view can be obtained from the subcostal, apical and parasternal window. We prefer the subcostal approach because of the excellent quality of the images obtained from this position. The ultrasonic beam reaches the heart more easily through the soft tissues from the subcostal area than through the chest wall from the other windows. The subcostal window allows better contact between skin and transducer, especially if slight pressure is applied. In addition, the great arteries can also be visualized when the ultrasonic beam is tilted from the four chamber view anteriorly. Compared with the other echo-windows ultrasound will pass more perpendicularly to the interatrial and the posterior interventricular septum which enhances the image quality of these structures. For a concise survey of the application of two-dimensional subcostal echocardiography in congenital heart disease the reader is referred to the work of Lange et al. (5). The apical approach of congenital heart disease is described by Silverman and Schiller (6). To obtain a parasternal four chamber view the ultrasonic beam should be rotated from the short axis position on mitral valve level slightly clockwise and tilted cranially. This view does not show the entire length of the ventricles and therefore it is called the parasternal foreshortened four chamber view (2).

A subcostal four chamber view is shown in Figure 1.17. The right ventricular inflow tract lies nearest to the transducer. The dorsal part of the tricuspid valve ring divides the right ventricle from the right atrium. The tricuspid valve leaflets should be looked for more anteriorly. On the left, and slightly posterior to the tricuspid valve, the mitral valve echo's are visualized. The inlet part of the interventricular septum can be seen. The atrial septum is clearly displayed and is continuous with the interventricular septum. Note the small but important difference between the level of the implantation of the mitral and the tricuspid valves into the interventricular septum. Compared with the mitral valve the tricuspid valve is attached closer to the apex of the heart. The small part of the interventricular septum between these two valves is referred to as the atrioventricular septum. It forms a partition between the right atrium and the left ventricle. The mitral valve is invariably situated in the left ventricle and the tricuspid valve in the right ventricle. Therefore, the level of implantation of these two valves is an important landmark for the anatomical differentiation of the two ventricles. The posterior wall of the left atrium is apparently interrupted by the entry of the pulmonary veins just above the mitral valve and near the dorsal end of the atrial septum. Behind the left atrium a transverse section of the descending aorta can be expected.

When the transducer is slightly tilted in a plane just superior and anterior to the four chamber view the left atrium and mitral valve will be replaced by the aorta and the aortic valve without altering the location of the right ventricle just above the transducer. This cross-section is referred to as the subcostal longitudinal view and visualizes the origin of the posterior great artery from the posteriorly located ventricle (Figure 1.18). If the plane of angulation is steep a transverse section of the main pulmonary artery becomes visible just to the left of the aorta. The course of the aorta may be traced by rotating the transducer in such a manner that the plane of cross-section coincides with that of the aortic arch. This plane will reveal the direction of the aortic arch. The interventricular septum, as seen in Figure 1.18, consists of the small membranous septum in the medial wall of the left ventricular outflow tract just below the aortic valve. The remaining muscular septum forms the

6

transitional zone between inlet and trabecular septum. The small echo within the right ventricle is probably caused by a small papillary muscle inserted into the interventricular septum. This identifies the anterior chamber as the anatomical right ventricle because the mitral valve has no septal insertions.

By exerting a little more pressure on the transducer and directing the ultrasonic beam from the subcostal longitudinal plane even more anteriorly the subcostal frontal view is obtained. As the name suggests it lies almost parallel to the frontal plane (Figure 1.19). In this plane the right ventricular outflow tract is bordered by the right atrium and the left ventricle. The anterior papillary muscle of the right ventricle is usually seen in transverse section. The pulmonary valve is often visible in the upper part of the sector. If the right ventricle is dilated the pulmonary valve will be particularly conspicuous (Figure 1.20). The main pulmonary artery is not visualized because of its sharp posterior angulation.

In summary we conclude that a) the parasternal long axis views (the long axis views of the right and left heart and the sagittal view through the main pulmonary artery and the descending aorta), b) the parasternal short axis views at different levels and c) the subcostal views (four chamber, longitudinal and frontal) are three echocardiographic approaches whereby all the structures of the heart and the great arteries are visualized. Therefore, these views should be routinely used. From the subcostal window additional information may be obtained when the transducer is rotated through 90° and the heart is scanned in a left to right or vice versa direction. This discloses the subcostal sagittal i.e. short axis views. Valuable information may also be obtained from the apical and suprasternal areas.

References

1. Bom N, Lancee CT, Van Zwieten G, Kloster FE, Roelandt J: Multi-scan echocardiography, I. Technical description. Circulation 48:1066 – 1074, 1973.
2. Tajik AJ, Seward JB, Hagler DJ, Mair DD, Lie JT: Two-dimensional real-time ultrasonic imaging of the heart and great vessels. Technique, image orientation, structure identification, and validation. Mayo Clin Proc 53:271 – 303, 1978.
3. Henry WL, DeMaria A, Gramiak R, King DL, Kisslo JA, Popp RL, Sahn DJ, Schiller NB, Tajik AJ, Teichholz LE, Weyman AE: Report of the American Society of Echocardiography committee on nomenclature and standards in two-dimensional echocardiography. Circulation 62:212 – 217, 1980.
4. Anderson RH: Embryology of the ventricular septum. In: Anderson RH, Shinebourne EA (eds.). Paediatric Cardiology 1977, Edinburgh, Churchill Livingstone, 1978, 103 – 112.
5. Lange LW, Sahn DJ, Allen HD, Goldberg SJ, Subxiphoid cross-sectional echocardiography in infants and children with congenital heart disease. Circulation 59:513 – 524, 1979.
6. Silverman NH, Schiller NB, Apex echocardiography. A two-dimensional technique for evaluating congenital heart disease. Circulation 57:503 – 511, 1978.

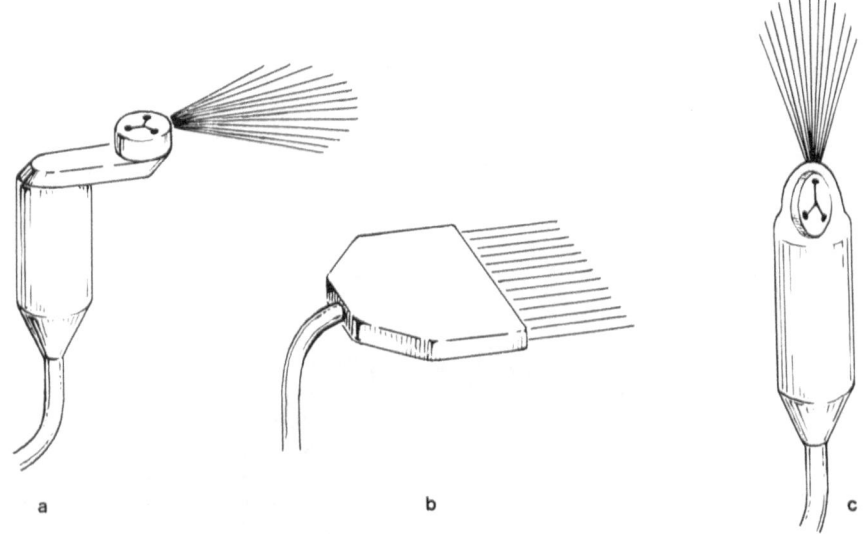

Figure 1.1. Diagrammatic drawings of the ATL mechanical sector scan transducer (a), the transducer of a linear array system (b) and an in-line scan head (c).

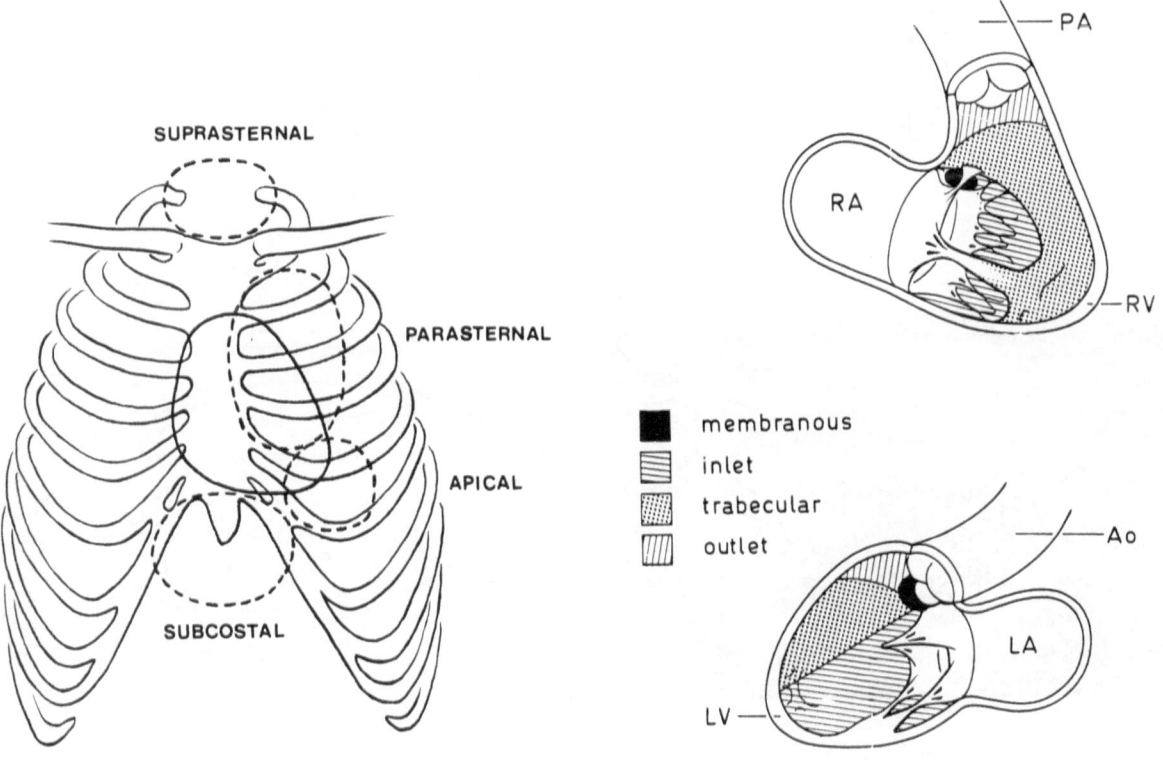

Figure 1.2. Illustration of the acoustic windows of the heart.

Figure 1.3. Diagrammatic representation of the right and left side of the interventricular septum, which is divided into its four parts.

PA = pulmonary artery, RA = right atrium, RV = right ventricle, Ao = aorta, LV = left ventricle, LA = left atrium.

8

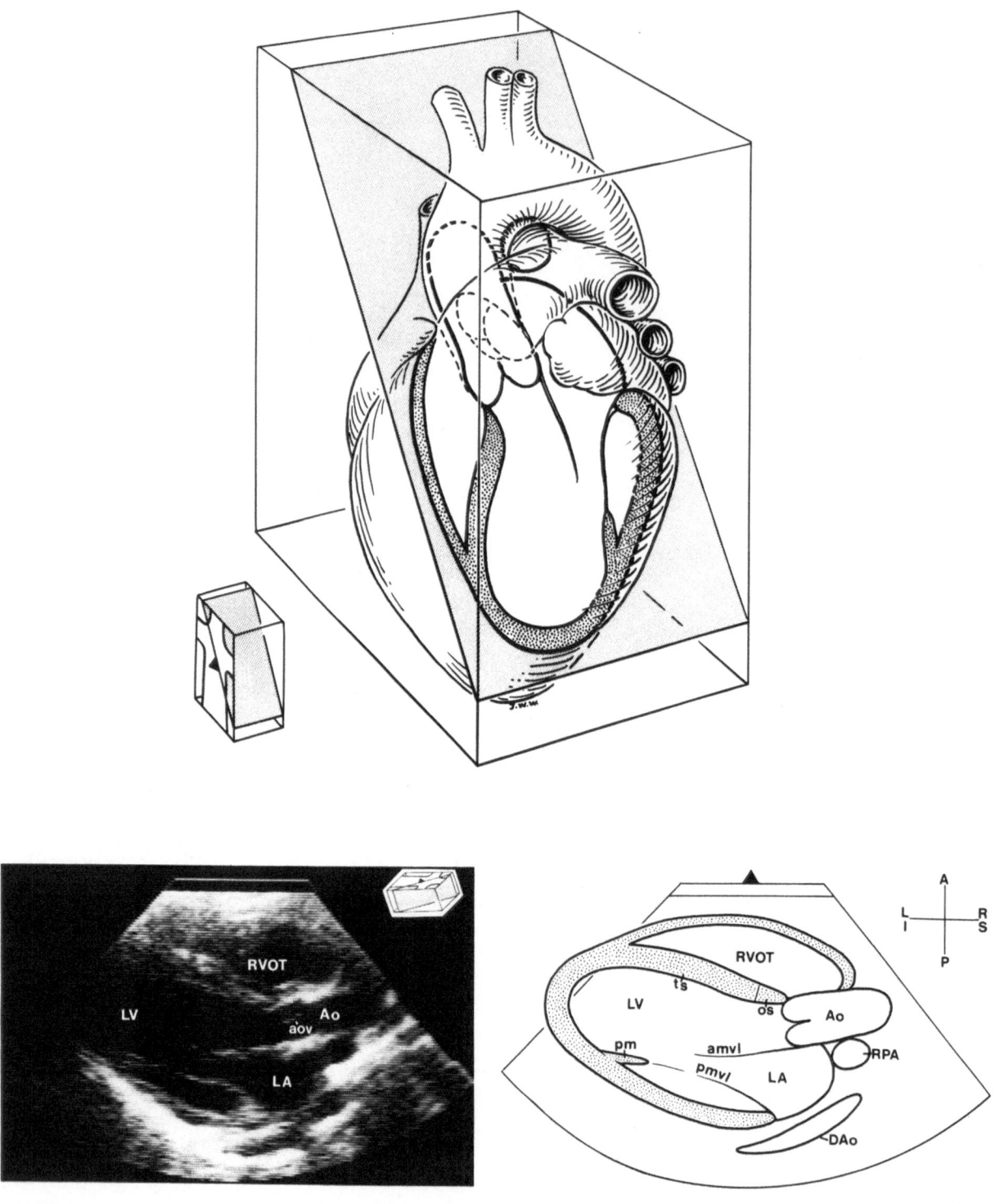

Figure 1.4. Parasternal long axis two-dimensional echocardiogram and diagrammatic drawings.

RVOT = right ventricular outflow tract. Ao = aorta, DAo = descending aorta, RPA = right pulmonary artery, LA = left atrium, LV = left ventricle, os = outlet septum, ts = trabecular septum, amvl = anterior mitral valve leaflet, pmvl = posterior mitral valve leaflet, pm = papillary muscle, aov = aortic valve, A = anterior, P = posterior, L = left, R = right, I = inferior, S = superior.

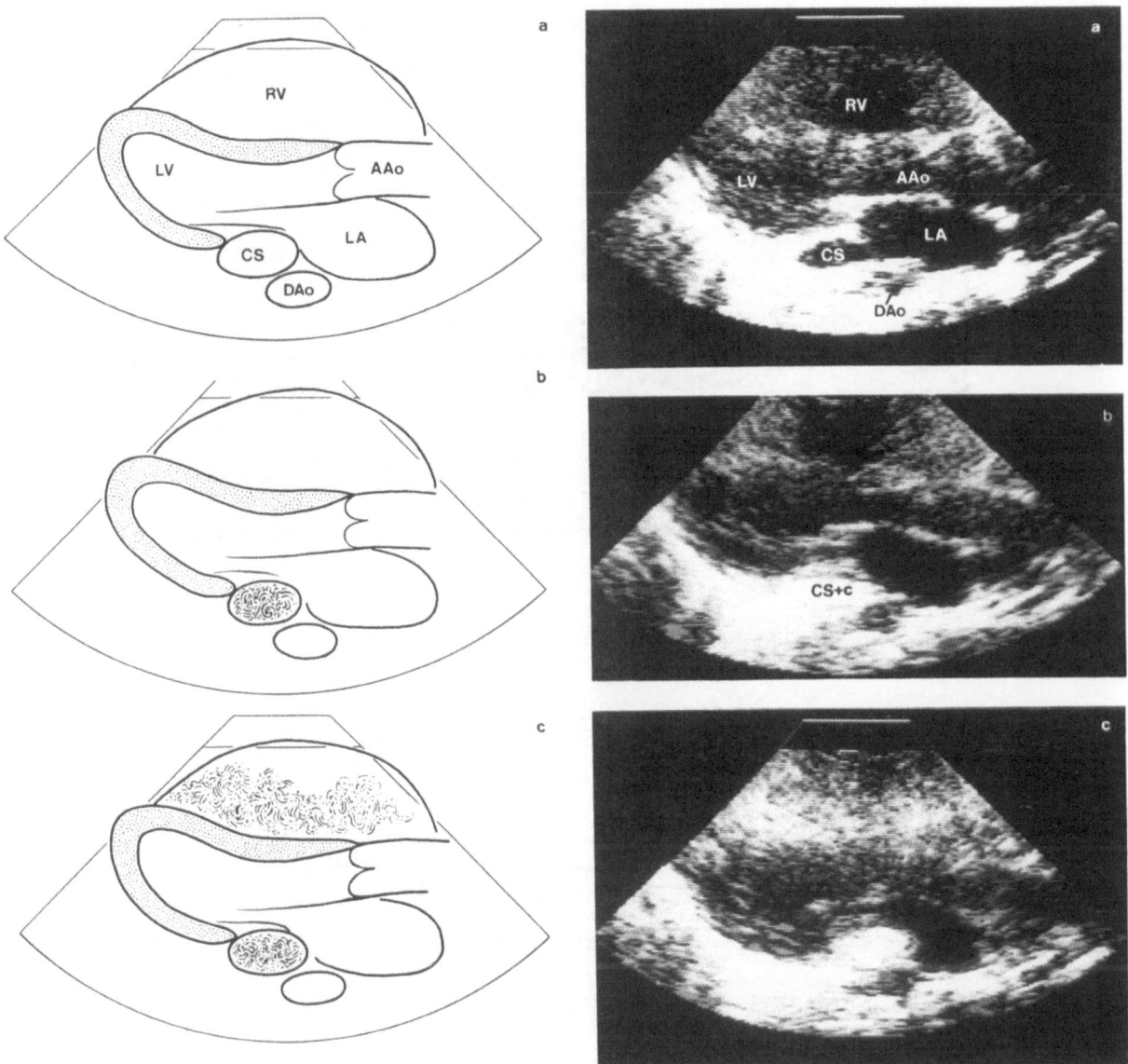

Figure 1.5. Parasternal long axis two-dimensional echocardiograms showing a transversely cut dilated coronary sinus in a patient with persistent left superior caval vein. A peripheral echocontrast (saline or 5% dextrose solution) injection into the left arm opacified the coronary sinus (b) and a moment later also the right ventricle (c).

RV = right ventricle, LV = left ventricle, LA = left atrium, AAo = ascending aorta. DAo = descending aorta, CS = coronary sinus, c = contrast.

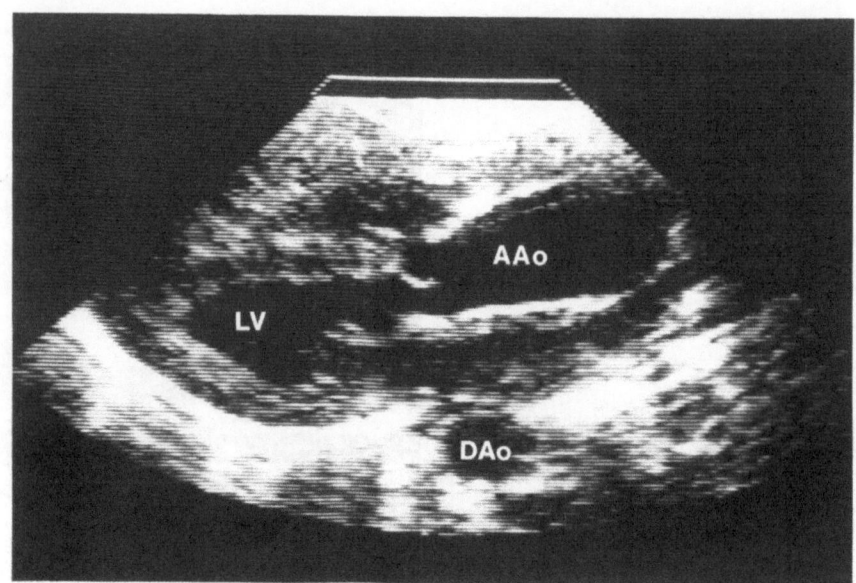

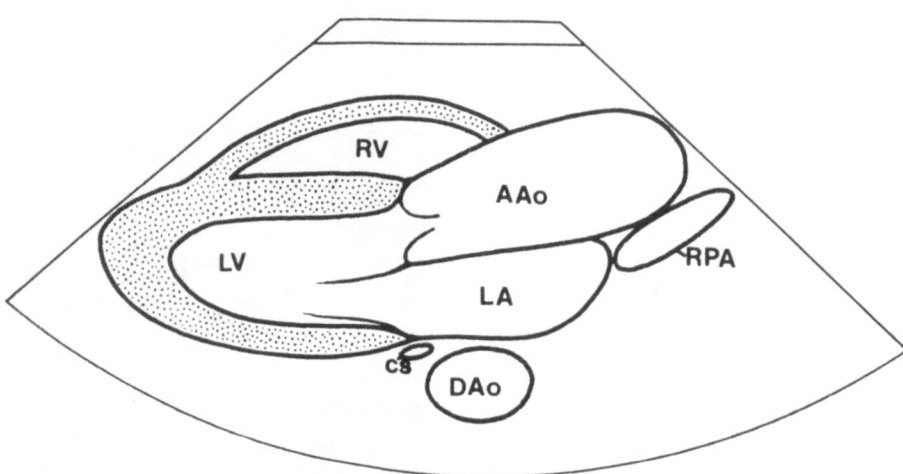

Figure 1.6. Parasternal long axis two-dimensional echocardiogram of a patient with a dilated ascending aorta.

RV = right ventricle, AAo = ascending aorta, LV = left ventricle, LA = left atrium, RPA = right pulmonary artery, cs = coronary sinus. DAo = descending aorta.

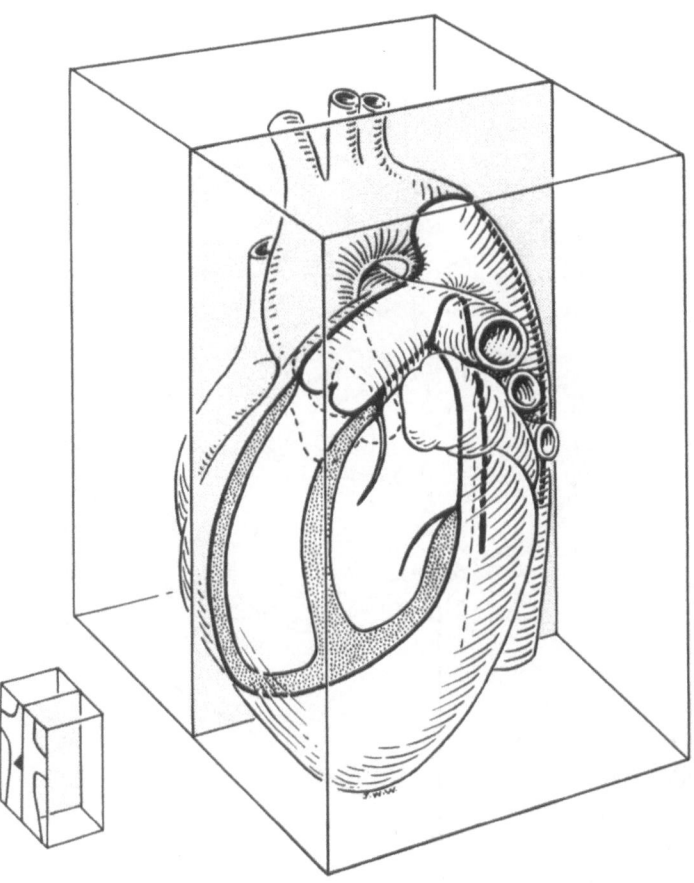

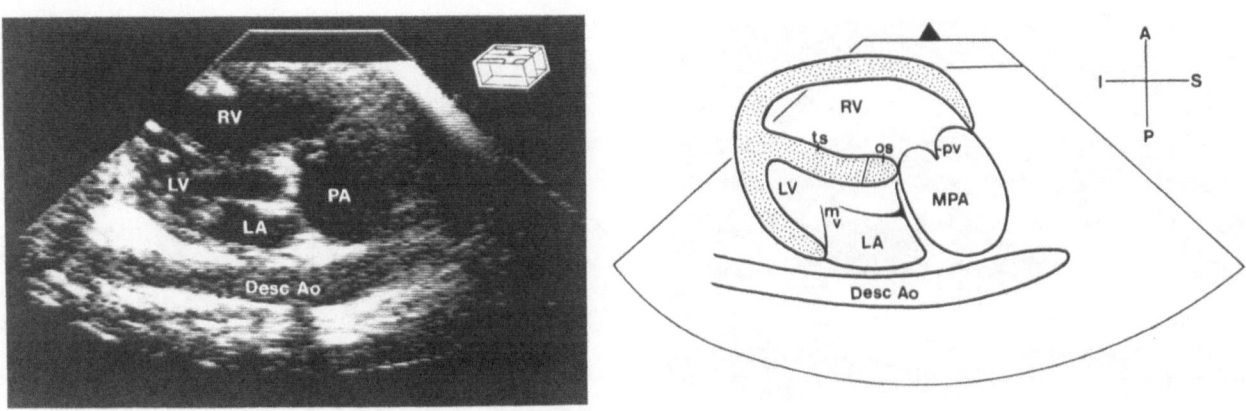

Figure 1.7. Parasternal sagittal two-dimensional echocardiogram through pulmonary artery and descending aorta.

RV = right ventricle, ts = trabecular septum, os = outlet septum, pv = pulmonary valve, MPA = main pulmonary artery, LV = left ventricle, LA = left atrium, mv = mitral valve, DescAo = descending aorta.

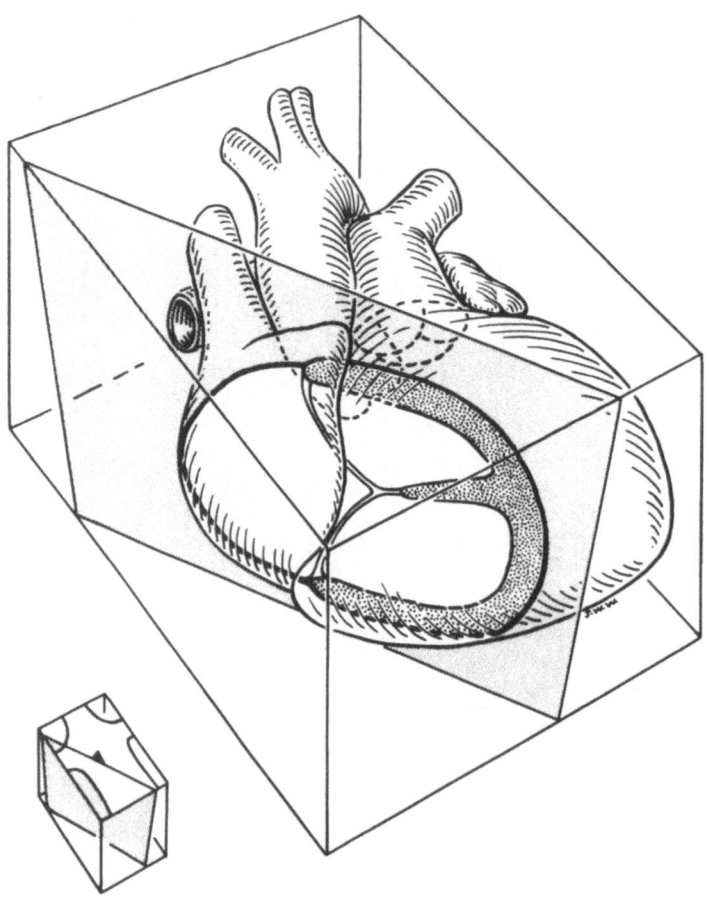

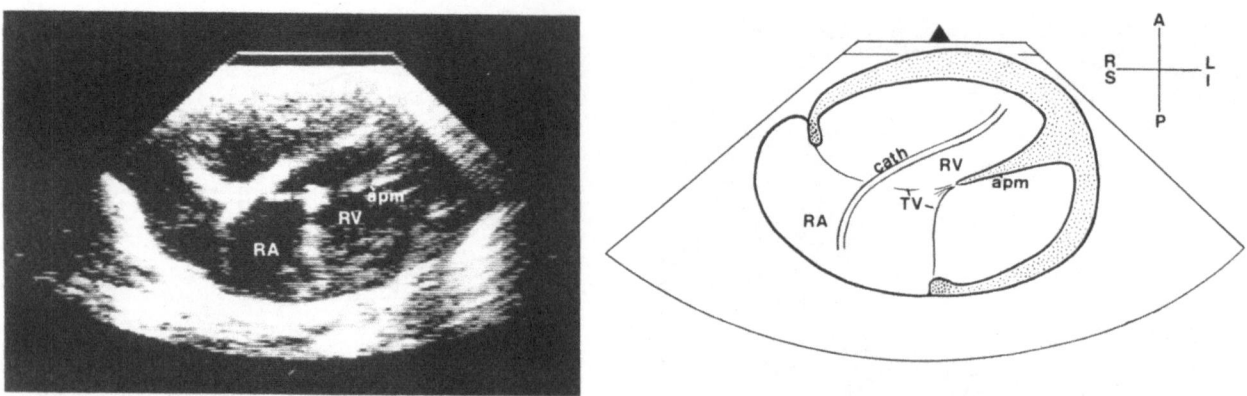

Figure 1.8. Parasternal long axis view of the right heart. The actual echocardiogram shows a catheter passing the tricuspid orifice from the right atrium into an anterior portion of the right ventricle.

RA = right atrium, TV = tricuspid valve, RV = right ventricle, apm = anterior papillary muscle, cath = catheter.

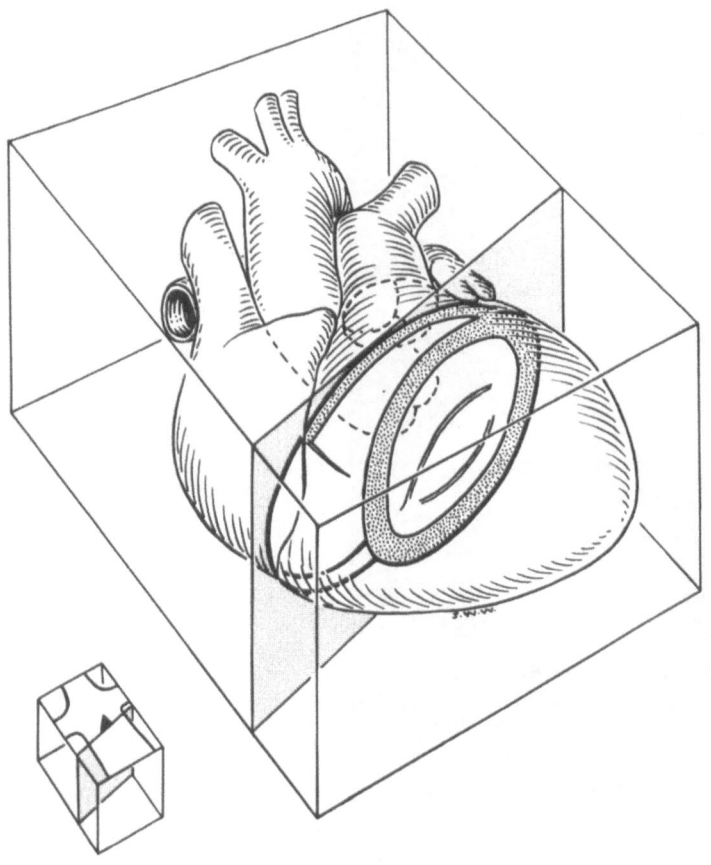

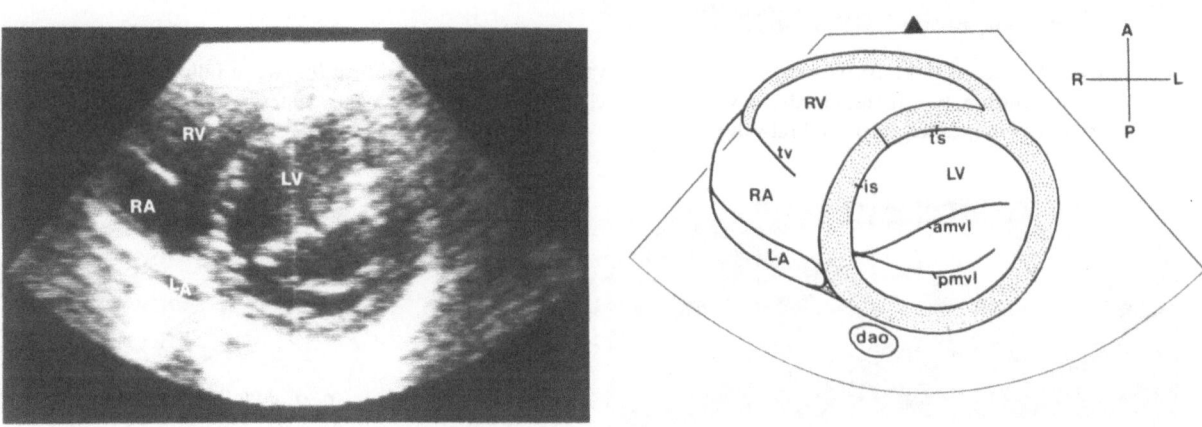

Figure 1.9. Parasternal short axis two-dimensional echocardiogram at the level of the mitral valve leaflets.

RV = right ventricle, tv = tricuspid valve, RA = right atrium, LA = left atrium, is = inlet septum, ts = trabecular septum, LV = left ventricle, amvl = anterior mitral valve leaflet, pmvl = posterior mitral valve leaflet, dao = descending aorta.

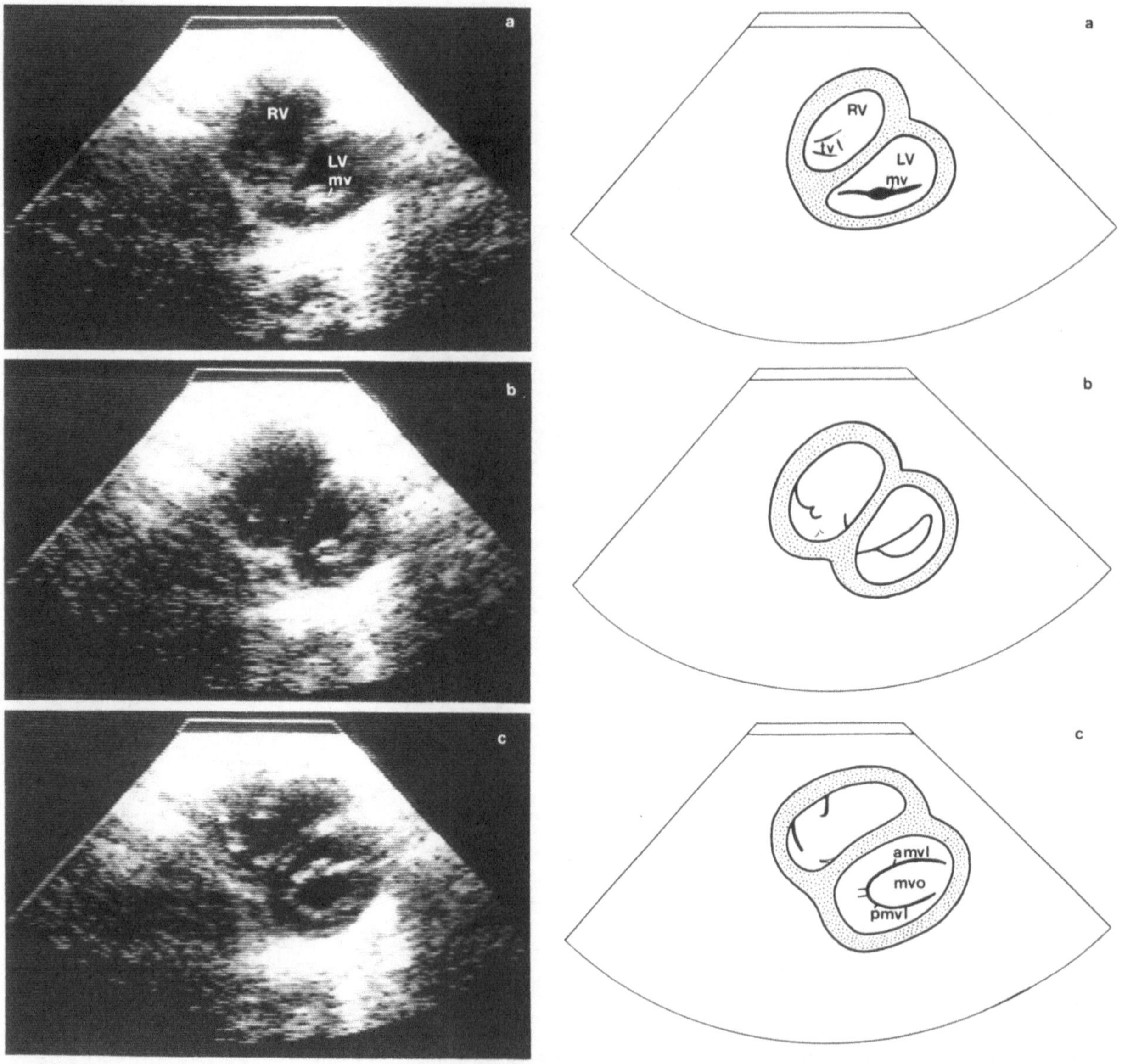

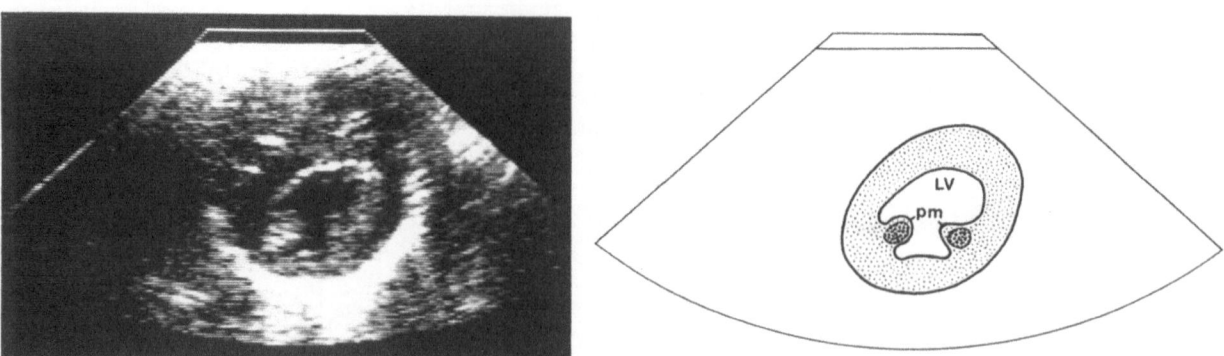

Figure 1.10. Parasternal short axis views showing the mitral valve closed (a), semi-opened (b) and in fully opened position (c).
RV = right ventricle, tv = tricuspid valve, LV = left ventricle, mv = mitral valve, amvl = anterior mitral valve leaflet, pmvl = posterior mitral valve leaflet, mvo = mitral valve orifice.

Figure 1.11. Parasternal short axis view on a lower level showing the papillary muscles in the left ventricle.
LV = left ventricle, pm = papillary muscle.

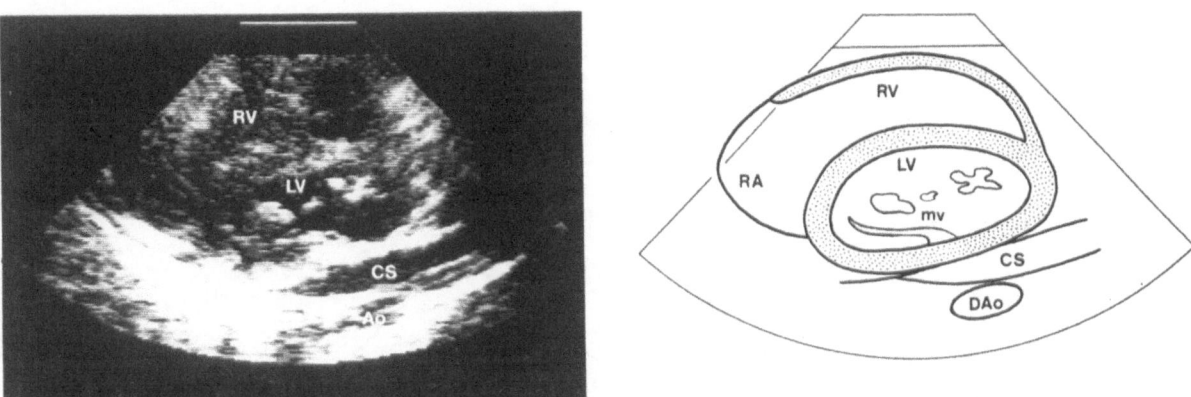

Figure 1.12. Parasternal short axis view demonstrating a longitudinal section through a dilated coronary sinus.

    RV = right ventricle, RA = right atrium, LV = left ventricle, mv = mitral valve, CS = coronary sinus, Ao = aorta, DAo = descending aorta.

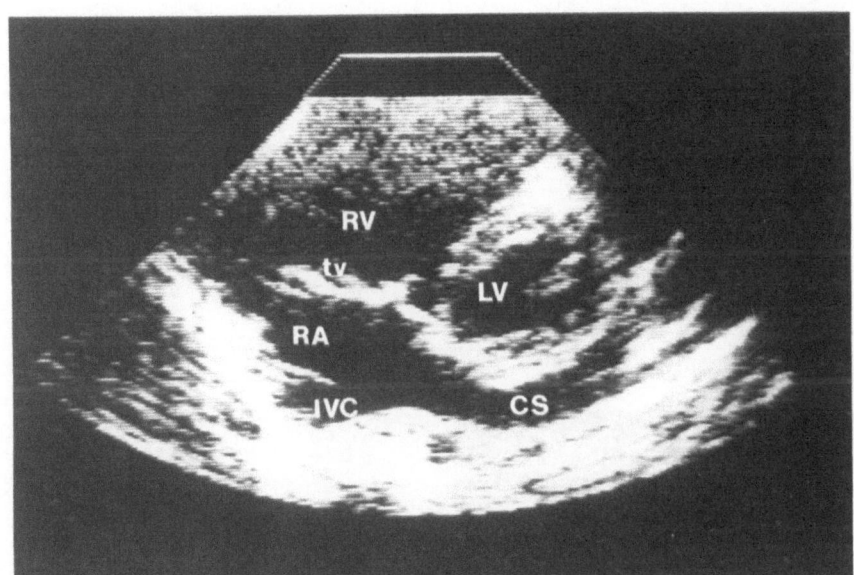

Figure 1.13. Parasternal short axis view of the same patient as in Figure 1.12. The drainage of the coronary sinus and inferior caval vein in the right atrium is visualized.

    RV = right ventricle, tv = tricuspid valve, RA = right atrium, LV = left ventricle, CS = coronary sinus, IVC = inferior vena cava.

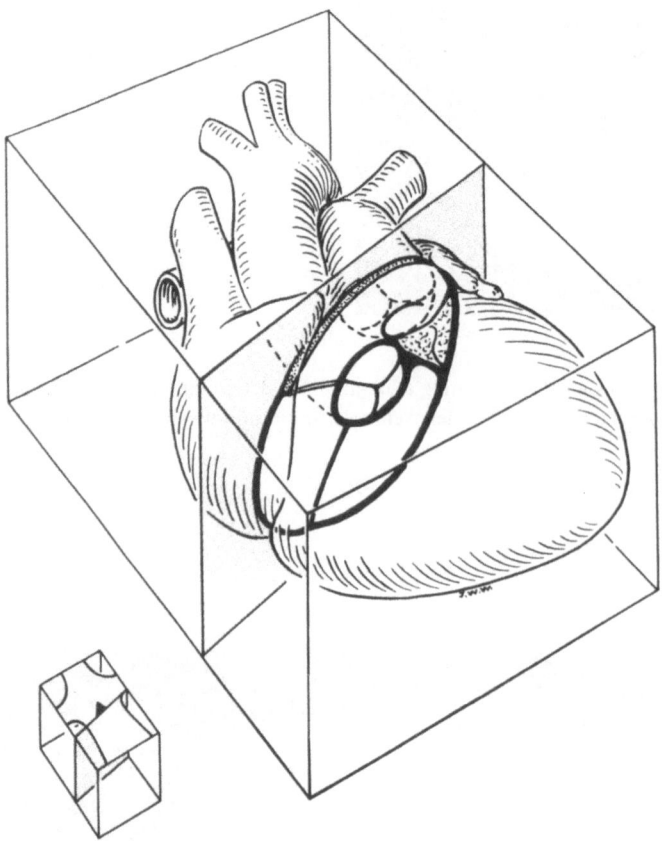

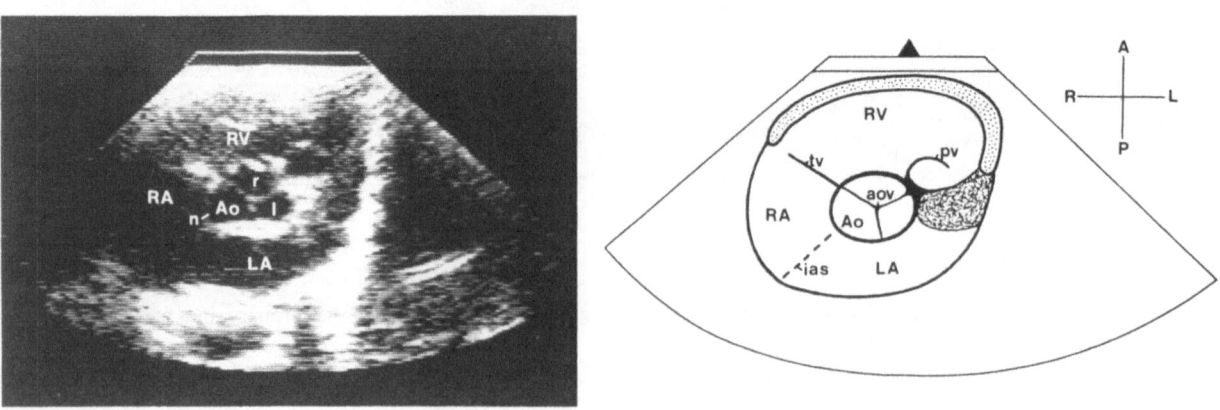

Figure 1.14. Parasternal short axis two-dimensional echocardiogram at the level of the semilunar valves.

RV = right ventricle, tv = tricuspid valve, RA = right atrium, ias = interatrial septum, LA = left atrium, pv = pulmonary valve. Ao = aorta, aov = aortic valve, r, l and n = right, left and non-coronary cusp.

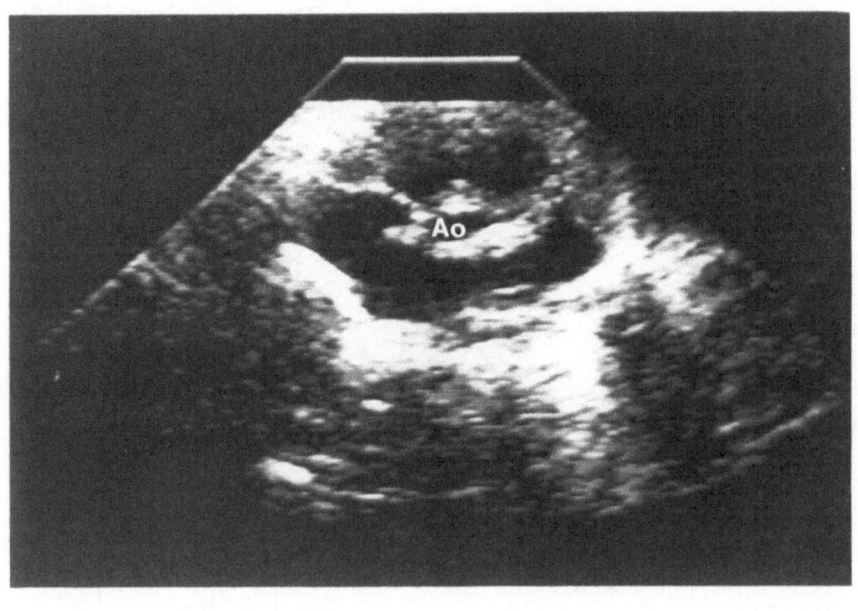

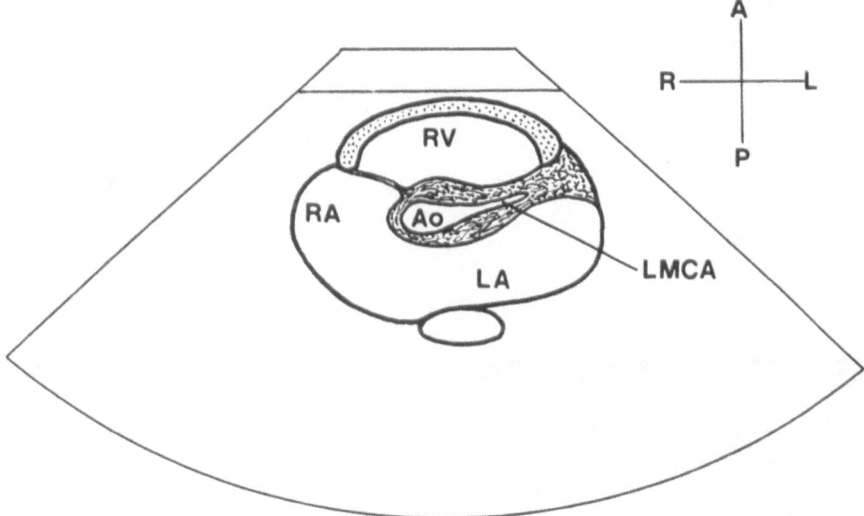

Figure 1.15. Parasternal short axis view showing the origin of the left main coronary artery from the aorta.
RA = right atrium, RV = right ventricle, Ao = aorta, LA = left atrium, LMCA = left main coronary artery.

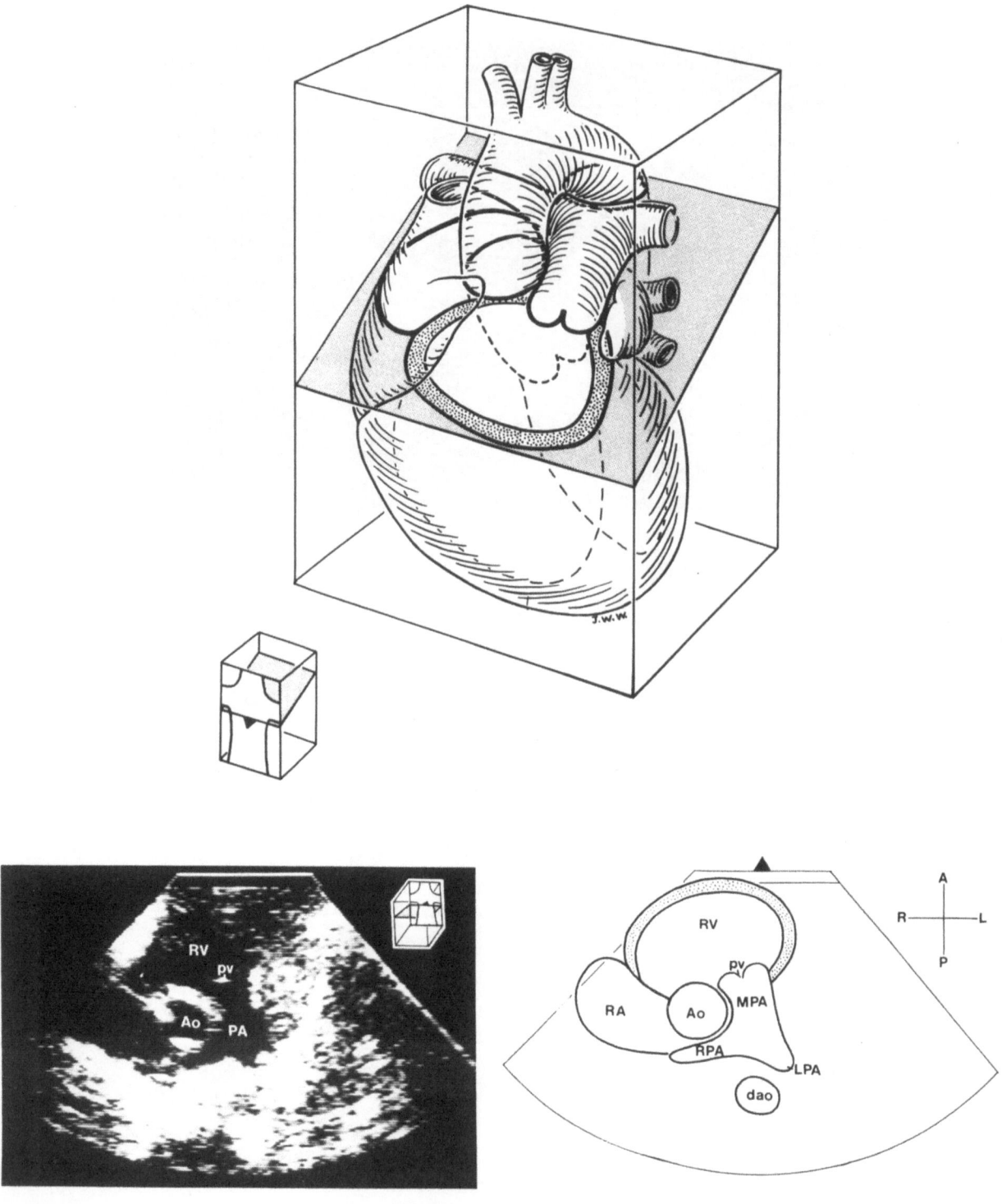

Figure 1.16. Parasternal short axis view at the level of the great arteries. The echocardiographic plane is slightly tilted cranially to visualize the bifurcation of the pulmonary artery.

RA = right atrium, RV = right ventricle, pv = pulmonary valve, MPA = main pulmonary artery, RPA = right pulmonary artery, LPA = left pulmonary artery, Ao = aorta, dao = descending aorta.

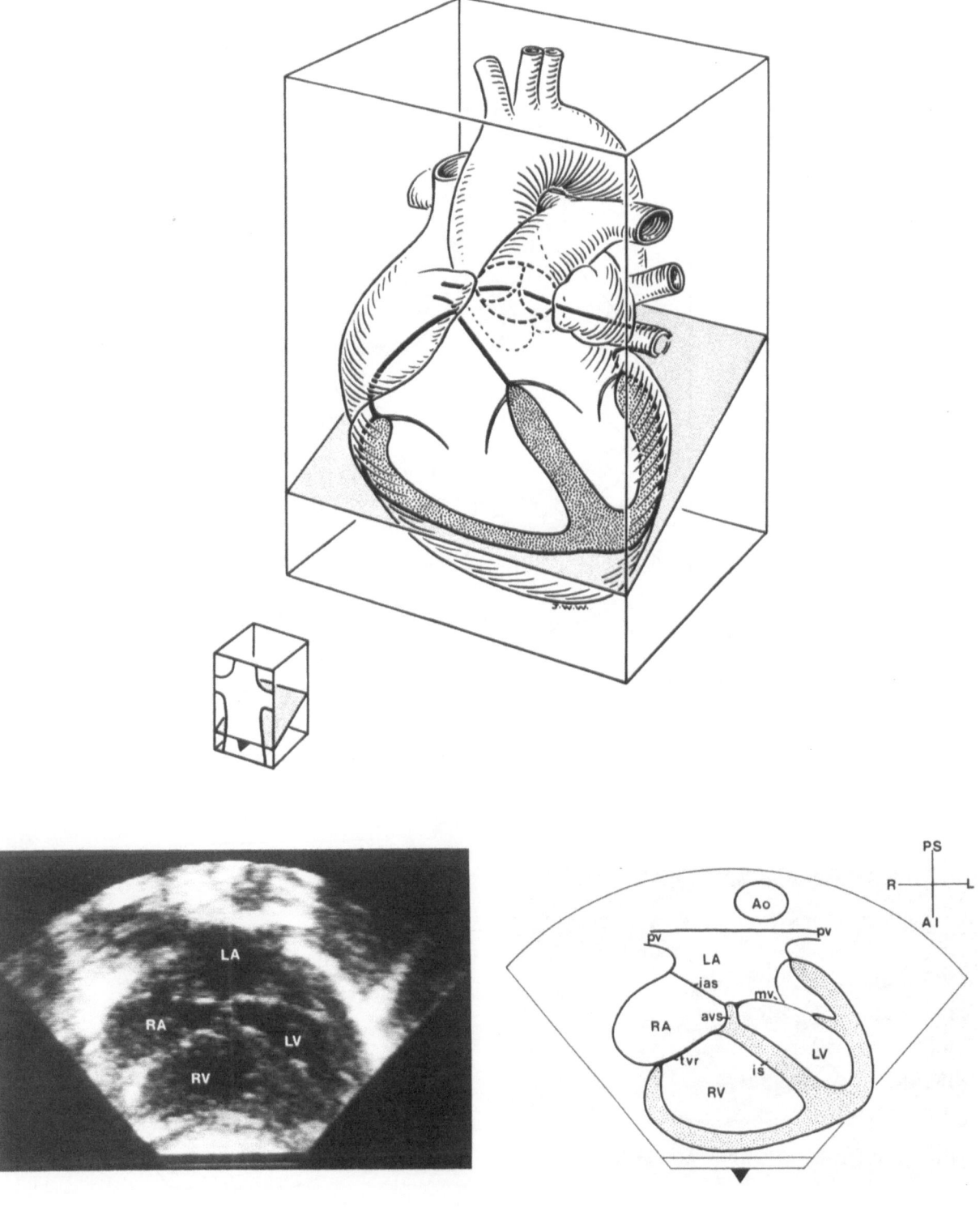

Figure 1.17. Subcostal four chamber two-dimensional echocardiogram. The heart in the diagrammatic chest shows tricuspid and mitral valve leaflets. In the actual echocardiogram only the tricuspid valve ring is visualized.

Ao = aorta, pv = pulmonary vein, ias = interatrial septum, LA = left atrium, RA = right atrium, mv = mitral valve, avs = atrioventricular septum, tvr = tricuspid valve ring, is = inlet septum, RV = right ventricle, LV = left ventricle.

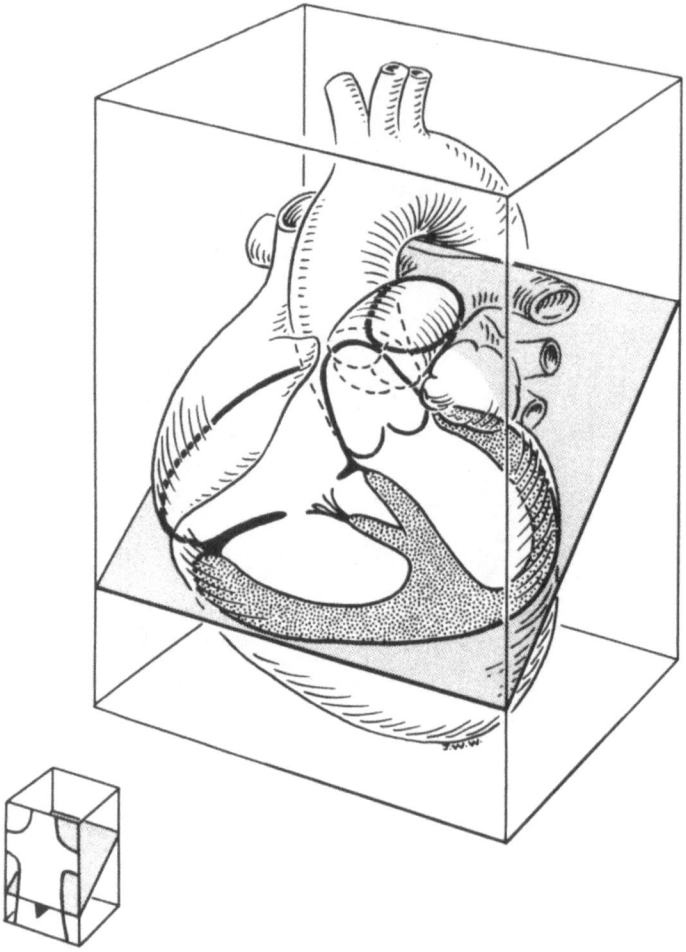

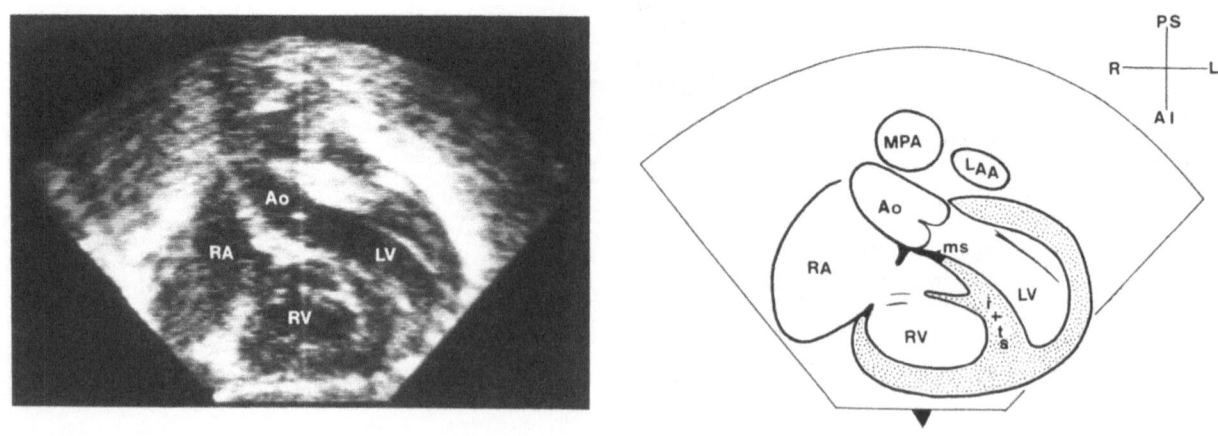

Figure 1.18. Subcostal longitudinal two-dimensional echocardiogram.

MPA = main pulmonary artery, LAA = left atrial appendage, Ao = aorta, RA = right atrium, RV = right ventricle, LV = left ventricle, ms = membranous septum, i + ts = transition zone between inlet- and trabecular septum.

21

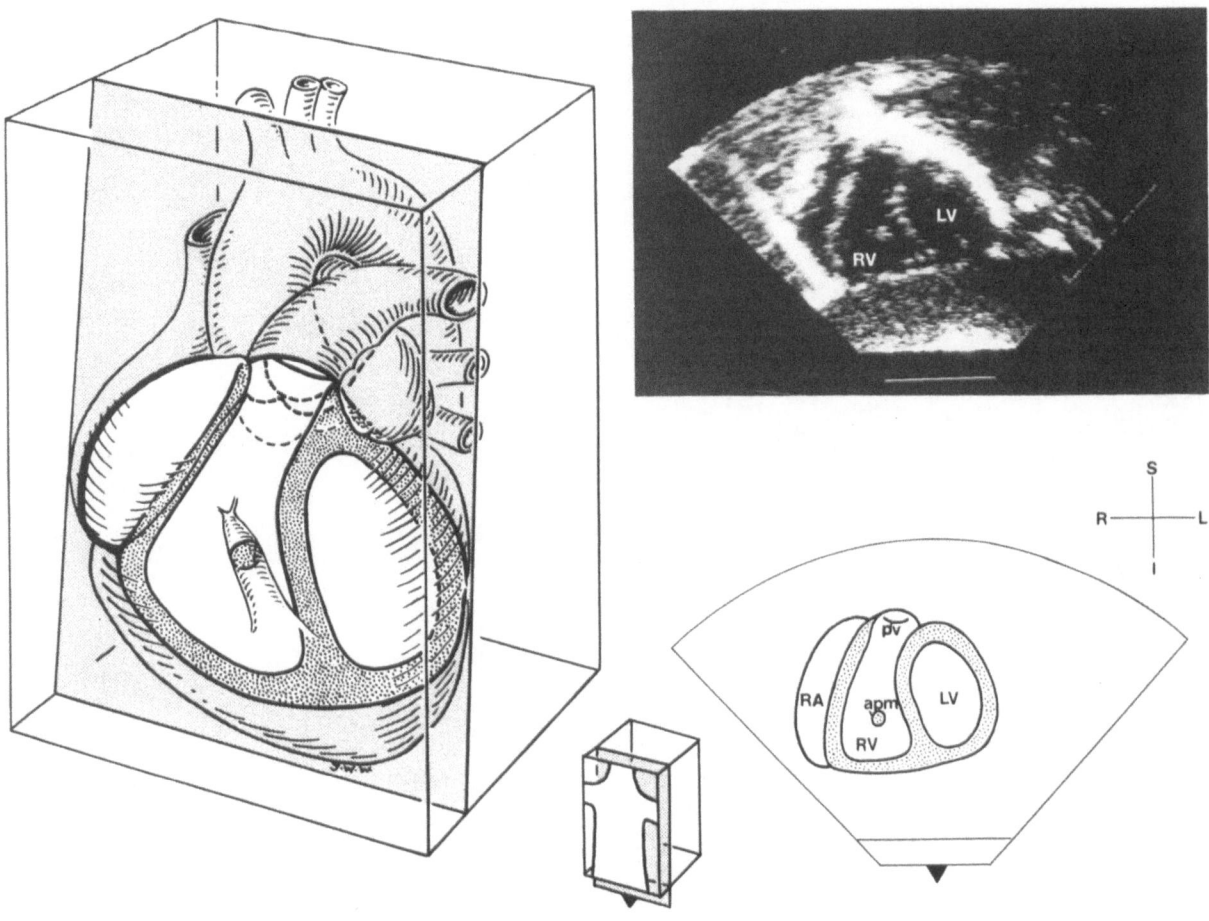

Figure 1.19. Subcostal frontal two-dimensional echocardiogram.
RA = right atrium, RV = right ventricle, LV = left ventricle, pv = pulmonary valve, apm = anterior papillary muscle.

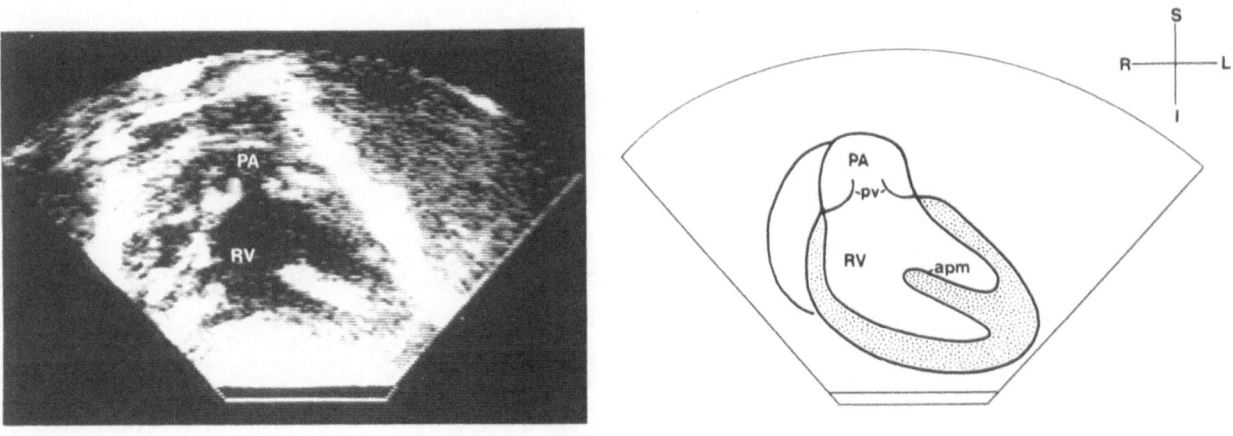

Figure 1.20. Subcostal frontal view in a case with dilated right ventricle.
pv = pulmonary valve leaflets, PA = pulmonary artery, RV = right ventricle, apm = anterior papillary muscle.

2. ISOLATED VENTRICULAR SEPTAL DEFECT

The ventricular septal defect is the most frequently occurring congenital cardiac defect. It may cause serious complaints in the first months of life. The pulmonary vascular resistance rapidly diminishes shortly after birth and the pressure in the right ventricle falls below that of the left ventricle. If there is an interventricular communication blood flows directly from the left into the right ventricle causing a volume overload of the pulmonary circulation and the left heart. The pulmonary artery pressure is related to the size of the defect and magnitude of the shunt. In the majority of the cases isolated ventricular septal defect can be diagnosed by physical examination, electrocardiogram and chest X-ray. The haemodynamic importance may be assessed to a certain extent by the antero-posterior diameter of the chest, the degree of dyspnoea, the duration of the systolic murmur, the intensity of the second heart sound and the presence or absence of a diastolic flow murmur. In addition, information may be acquired from the cardiac size and pulmonary plethora on the chest X-ray. Additional quantitative information on the magnitude of the L-R shunt can be obtained from the M-mode echocardiogram which allows accurate measurements of the left atrial and the left ventricular dimensions. Particularly important to the pediatric cardiologist is the group of patients with isolated ventricular septal defect which develops cardiac failure with feeding problems and failure to thrive in the first months of life. These patients have large defects and often require corrective surgery. Some patients with a large ventricular septal defect, however, have few complaints and few clinical signs, erroneously suggesting a small defect. Nonetheless, they may develop a high pulmonary vascular resistance. Therefore, it is essential that all patients with a ventricular septal defect are submitted to an early complete non-invasive cardiac investigation to assess the severity of the lesion. Large ventricular septal defects can readily be visualized by two-dimensional echocardiography (1, 2, 3, 4). They appear as a distinct interruption of the normal continuity of the interventricular septum. On the relevant cross-sections they can be localized and their extension into the septum accurately identified.

As explained in chapter 1 the interventricular septum can be divided into four components. The inlet, trabecular and outlet parts of the muscular septum converge to the membranous septum. These four components of the interventricular septum are diagrammatically shown in the routinely used echocardiographic cross-sections in Figure 2.1. The classification of the different types of defects used in this atlas is based on that proposed by Moulaert (5) and subsequently modified by Soto and associates (6). See Table 2.1. Large defects are never confined to the relatively small membranous septum alone but always extend into the muscular part of the septum, hence the introduction of the concept perimembranous ventricular septal defect. In this concept three types are recognized according to their manner of extension into the three

Table 2.1. Classification of ventricular septal defects

Type	Subcategories
Perimembranous	– inlet (posterior)
	– trabecular
	– outlet (infundibular)
Muscular	– inlet
	– trabecular
	– outlet
Subarterial outlet	

Mixed and multiple defects.

components of the muscular septum. Also, as a consequence of the division of the muscular septum, we distinguish three types of pure muscular defects. In these defects the membranous septum remains intact and the circumference of the defects is always comprised of muscular tissue. The subarterial outlet defect is localized at the extreme superior position so that it borders the semilunar valve rings. Therefore, the circumference of this type of defect does not entirely consist of muscular tissue. The different types of ventricular septal defect will be discussed according to their location and extension.

Perimembranous ventricular septal defect

The drawing of Figure 2.2 corresponds with the echocardiograms of Figure 2.4 and Figure 2.5. The subcostal longitudinal view in these figures displays simultaneously the septal tricuspid leaflet and the aortic valve. A ventricular septal defect is situated at the site of the membranous septum, i.e. in the medial wall of the left ventricular outflow tract directly beneath the aortic valve. When viewed from the right side the defect is located just inferior to the attachment of the septal leaflet of the tricuspid valve. This defect was not visualized in the four chamber view nor in the parasternal views indicative of a limited extension. Larger defects are seen at corresponding sites of the interventricular septum in different cross-sections. In these cases there is no doubt as to the presence, location and size of the defect. If the defect is seen in only one cross-section its presence can be proven only during the actual real time imaging. The defect should be continuously observed while the remaining part of the interventricular septum is accurately visualized. Several important phenomena should be appreciated. The size of the defect may vary during the cardiac cycle, whereby the defect is larger in diastole than in systole (3). In the authors' experience haemodynamically important defects do not close completely during systole. During the movements of the heart the ventricular septal defect may disappear from the echocardiographic plane. This is particularly liable to occur during visualization of the perimembranous type in the parasternal short axis view. Therefore, subcostal

views are preferred. A perimembranous ventricular septal defect may be covered from the right side by the septal leaflet of the tricuspid valve thus masking the defect, particularly during diastole. An important aid in detecting a ventricular septal defect is the presence of a bright echospot at the edge of the defect (Figure 2.3). Canale et al. (3) called this broadening of septal edges around a ventricular septal defect a T-artefact.

To avoid false positive findings only standard views, which clearly visualize both ventricles with the interventricular septum, should be used.

Additional echocardiographic information can be obtained during cardiac catheterization. The actual discontinuity of the interventricular septum can be passed by a cardiac catheter (Figure 2.4). Injection of echocontrast (saline or 5% dextrose solution) (7) into the left ventricle will reveal the actual L-R shunt. The echocontrast should clearly opacify the defect and pass into the contralateral ventricle (Figure 2.5). To reveal a R-L shunt echocontrast injection into a peripheral vein may suffice. The direction of flow should also be noticed. For instance, the two-dimensional echocardiograms in Figure 2.5 clearly show that the contrast enters the right ventricle in a superior to inferior direction, corresponding with the high localization of the defect. Inferior to superior flows of contrast into the right ventricle after left ventricular contrast injection are compatible with muscular defects situated in the inferior part of the septum.

Another echocontrast study to identify ventricular septal defects, recommended by some authors, is the negative contrast technique (8).

Figure 2.6 demonstrates a ventricular septal defect in different cross-sections. The subcostal longitudinal view exhibits a large subaortic defect in the region of the membranous septum. Several septal insertions of the tricuspid valve cover the defect at this level. The four chamber view shows a distinct deficiency of the upper part of the inlet septum including the atrioventricular septum as indicated by the arrow. With angulation of the transducer from the subcostal longitudinal view to the subcostal four chamber view the defect in the region of the membranous septum was seen to be clearly continuous with the defect in the inlet septum. In the short axis view the defect is on the right side of the left ventricular outflow tract. The anterior extension of the defect was restricted, therefore it was not visualized in the long axis view (not exhibited here). This defect can be classified as a perimembranous inlet defect previously described as the isolated common atrioventricular canal type defect (9). It is of surgical importance to differentiate between this type and the pure muscular inlet septal defect. In the latter the conduction system of the heart lies anteriorly to the defect, whereas it lies posteriorly to the perimembranous inlet defect.

During and after spontaneous closure of a perimembranous defect an aneurysm of the membranous septum may be present which can be visualized by two-dimensional echocardiography (10, 11) (Figure 2.7).

Muscular inlet ventricular septal defect

The two-dimensional echocardiograms of a muscular inlet septal defect are shown in Figure 2.8. In the subcostal longitudinal view the membranous septum is intact. The anterior part of the interventricular septum, visualized in the long axis view, is also intact. In the four chamber view a large defect is present in the upper part of the inlet septum between the septal leaflets of the tricuspid and mitral valves. In the short axis view at the level of the mitral valve, the defect is seen in the corresponding posterior part of the septum. Another example of an inlet septal defect is shown in the four chamber view of Figure 2.9. The subcostal longitudinal view of this case differentiates this septal deficiency from a perimembranous defect. The actual membranous septum here is intact. A marked deficiency is seen at the junction of the inlet and trabecular septa. Therefore, this is an example of a combination of a large pure muscular inlet and trabecular defect. Figure 2.10 exhibits the two-dimensional echocardiograms of a patient with two defects in the muscular inlet septum. The subcostal four chamber and longitudinal views show a muscular inlet defect extending into the trabecular septum. In the short axis view, at the level of the mitral valve, two defects are visible, a small anterior and a larger posterior defect. In the *other short* axis view (right and below) the

transducer is shifted to the apex of the heart. The defects remain in view suggesting the presence of two slit-like oblong deficiencies.

Muscular trabecular ventricular septal defect

The trabecular ventricular septal defect is situated in the trabecular part of the interventricular septum adjoining the inlet portion. The two-dimensional echocardiogram of a patient with this type of defect is shown in Figure 2.11. The long axis view exhibits a large anteriorly and apically located septal deficiency. In the short axis view the posterior part of the interventricular septum is intact. The defect is localized in the anterior trabecular portion where it joins the inlet septum. In the subcostal longitudinal view and the subcostal four chamber view (not exhibited here) the membranous septum and the inlet septum were clearly intact. The trabecular defect can occur as an isolated lesion but it is often associated with coarctation of the aorta. Figure 2.12 displays another left ventricular contrast injection in a case with a trabecular septal defect in the short axis view (a). The contrast opacifies the left ventricle and the defect (b) and passes through it into the right ventricle (c).

Muscular outlet ventricular septal defect

Figure 2.13 shows the two-dimensional echocardiogram of a patient with a ventricular septal defect and pulmonary hypertension. The long axis view exhibits a large defect of the outlet septum just beneath the aortic valve. The anterior wall of the aorta is located more anteriorly than the interventricular septum, which indicates some degree of overriding. This outlet defect is also known as the Fallot-like ventricular septal defect.

Subarterial outlet ventricular septal defect

Figure 2.14 shows the two-dimensional echocardiograms of an outlet defect in the subpulmonary, supracristal area. This type of defect is denoted by the authors, according to the classification describ-

26

ed earlier, as the subarterial outlet ventricular septal defect. In the long axis view the defect is located at the level of the aortic valve. One can imagine that the extreme superior location of the defect easily allows a prolapse of the right coronary cusp of the aortic valve through the defect, which can be detected in the long axis view (12). In the short axis view the defect is on the left side of the aortic ring in close relationship to the pulmonary valve. The sagittal view also shows the close relationship between the defect and the pulmonary valve. A venous echocontrast study in this patient revealed a R-L shunt through the defect due to the presence of pulmonary hypertension (Figure 2.15).

Determination of the exact location and extension of trabecular and outlet defects may influence the surgical approach. Sometimes these defects can be closed through the transatrial approach. However, the more distant the defect is situated from the tricuspid orifice the more likely the need for a ventriculotomy.

Multiple ventricular septal defects

When a ventricular septal defect is seen in different cross-sections but at non-corresponding sites more than one defect should be suspected. Careful analysis may reveal whether or not these defects communicate which each other. In the 'Swiss cheese' ventricular septal defect the many smaller communications cannot be visualized directly, they are hidden between or behind the many trabeculations. Left ventricular echocontrast injections are needed to identify these defects.

References

1. Cheatham JP, Latson LA, Gutgesell HP: Ventricular septal defect in infancy. Detection with two-dimensional echocardiography. Am J Card 47:85 – 89, 1981.
2. Bierman FZ, Fellows K, Williams RG: Prospective identification of ventricular septal defects in infancy using subxiphoid two-dimensional echocardiography. Circulation 62:807 – 817, 1980.
3. Canale JM, Sahn DJ, Allen HD, Goldberg SJ, Valdes-Cruz LM, Ovitt TW: Factors affecting real-time, cross-sectional echocardiographic imaging of perimembranous ventricular septal defects. Circulation 63:689 – 697, 1981.
4. Sutherland GR, Godman MJ, Smallhorn JF, Guiterras P, Anderson RH: Ventricular septal defects. Two-dimensional echocardiographic and morphological correlations. Br Heart J 47:316 – 328, 1982.
5. Moulaert AJ: Anatomy of ventricular septal defect. In: Anderson RH, Shinebourne EA (eds.). Paediatric Cardiology 1977, Edinburgh, Churchill Livingstone, 1978, 113 – 124.
6. Soto B, Becker AE, Moulaert AJ, Lie JT, Anderson RH: Classification of isolated ventricular septal defects. Br Heart J 43:332 – 343, 1980.
7. Gramiak RT, Shah PM, Kramer DH: Ultrasound cardiography. Contrast studies in anatomy and function. Radiology 92:939, 1969.
8. Funabashi T, Yoshida H, Nakaya S, Maeda T, Taniguchi N: Echocardiographic visualization of ventricular septal defect in infants and assessment of hemodynamic status using a contrast technique. Circulation 64:1025 – 1031, 1981.
9. Neufeld NH, Titus JL, Dushane JW, Burchell HB, Edwards JE: Isolated ventricular septal defect of the persistent common atrioventricular canal type. Circulation 23:685 – 696, 1961.
10. Snider AR, Silverman NH, Schiller NB, Ports TA: Echocardiographic evaluation of ventricular septal aneurysms. Circulation 59:920 – 926, 1979.
11. Canale JM, Sahn DJ, Valdes-Cruz LM, Allen HD, Goldberg SJ, Ovitt TW: Accuracy of two-dimensional echocardiography in the detection of aneurysms of the ventricular septum. Am Heart J 101:255 – 259, 1981.
12. Aziz KU, Cole RB, Paul MH: Echocardiographic features of supracristal ventricular septal defect with prolapsed aortic valve leaflet. Am J Card 43:854 – 859, 1979.

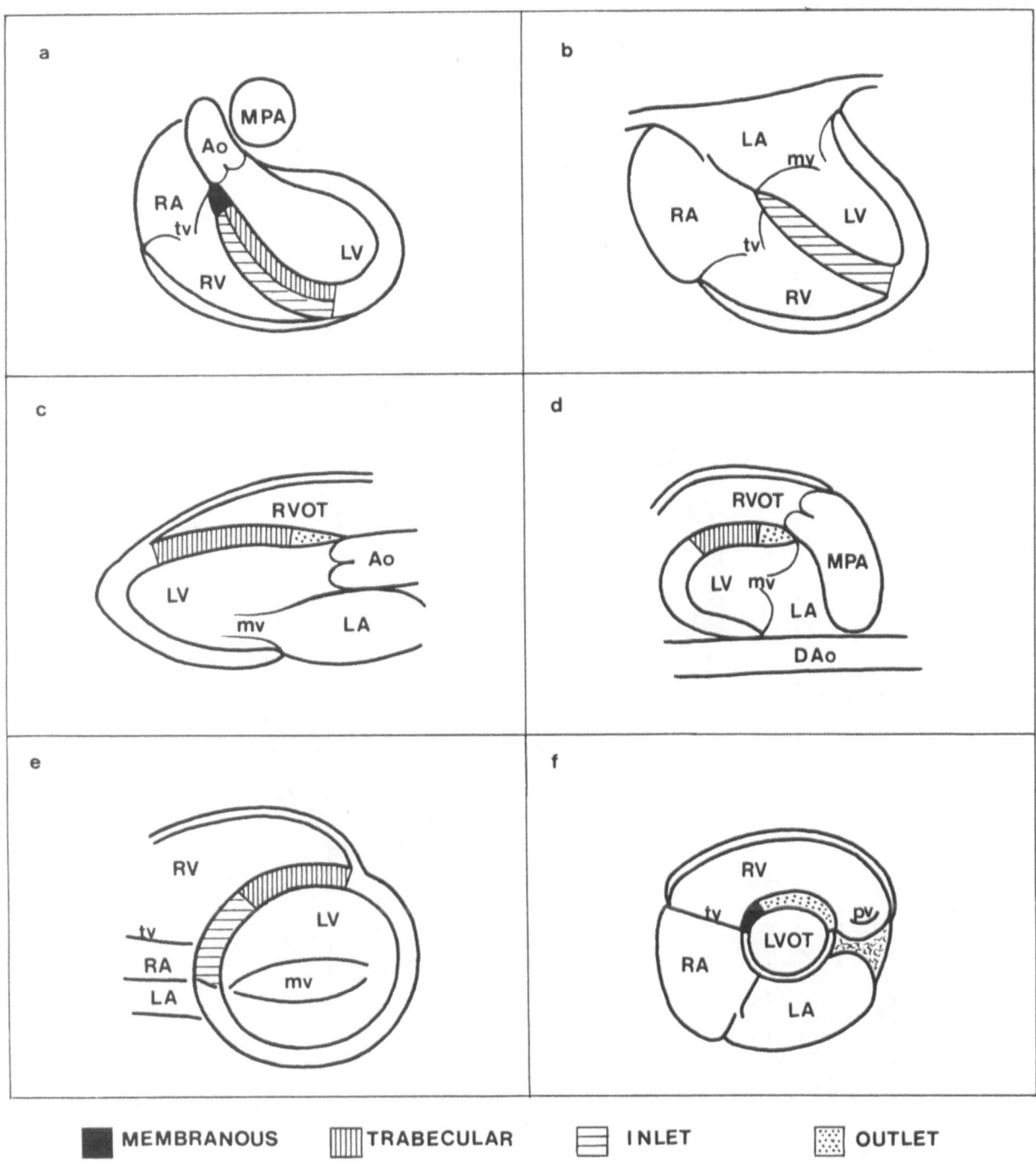

MEMBRANOUS   TRABECULAR   INLET   OUTLET

Figure 2.1. Diagrammatic representation of the matching cross-sectional planes showing the different components of the interventricular septum. The subcostal longitudinal view (a) exhibits the membranous septum and the transition zone between the inlet and trabecular septa. The four chamber view (b) only shows the muscular inlet septum. The small part between the attachments of the tricuspid and mitral valves is the atrioventricular septum. In the parasternal long axis view (c) and the parasternal sagittal view through the pulmonary artery (d) the trabecular and outlet septa are visualized. In the short axis view on mitral valve level (e) the trabecular septum is anterior and the inlet septum posterior. In the short axis view through the left ventricular outflow tract (f) the membranous septum is just anterior to the tricuspid valve attachment, the remaining part consists of outlet septum.

Ao = aorta, MPA = main pulmonary artery, RA = right atrium, RV = right ventricle, LV = left ventricle, tv = tricuspid valve, LA = left atrium, mv = mitral valve, RVOT = right ventricular outflow tract, DAo = descending aorta, LVOT = left ventricular outflow tract, pv = pulmonary valve.

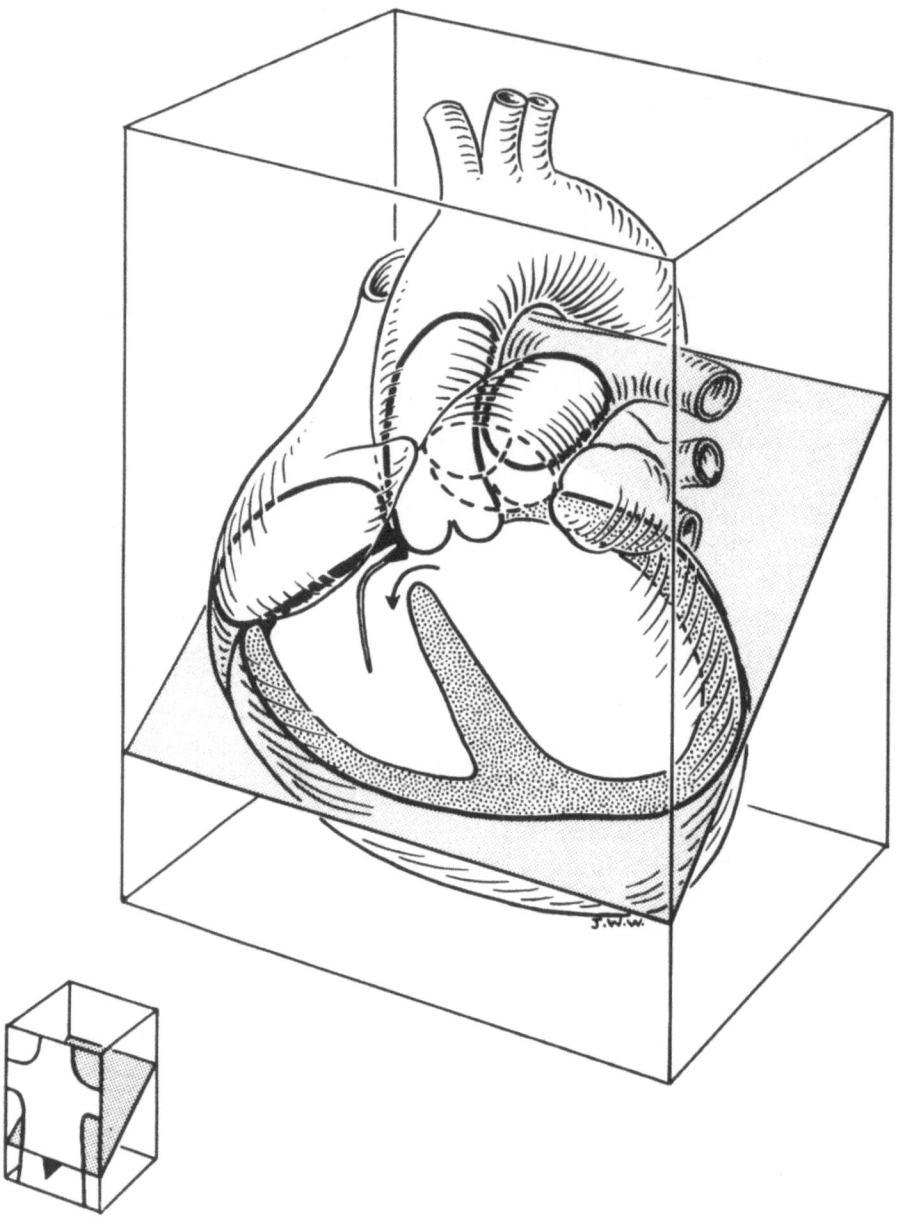

Figure 2.2. Diagrammatic representation of the subcostal longitudinal view exhibiting a membranous ventricular septal defect (arrow).

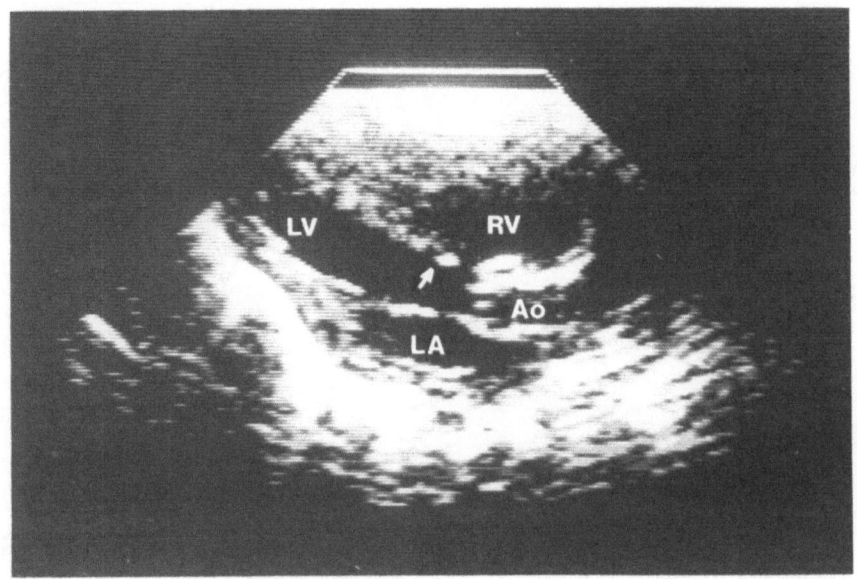

Figure 2.3. Parasternal long axis two-dimensional echocardiogram of a patient with a ventricular septal defect. There is a septal deficiency in the subaortic region. The inferior rim of the defect shows a bright echospot (arrow).

LV = left ventricle, RV = right ventricle, LA = left atrium, Ao = aorta.

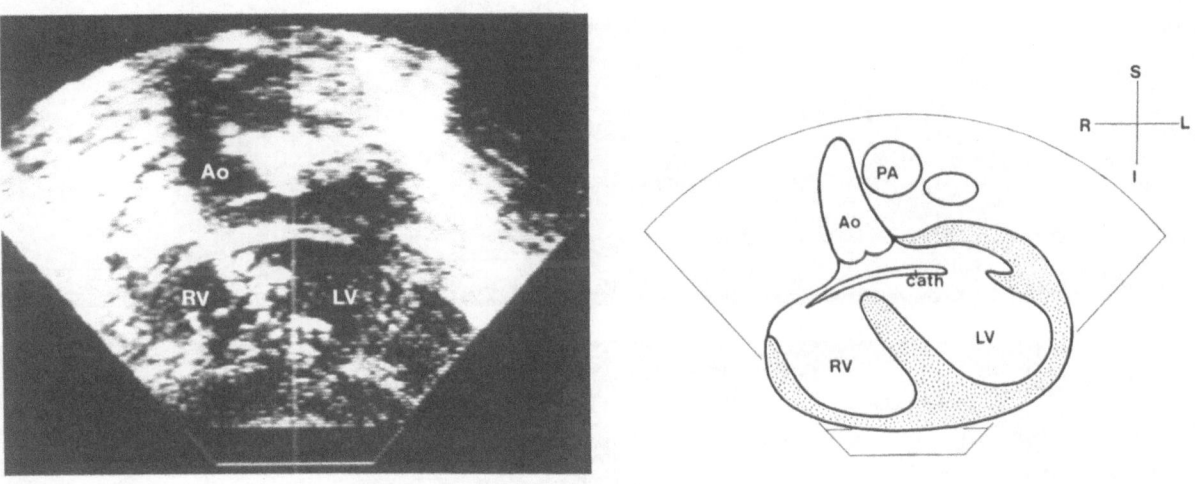

Figure 2.4. Subcostal longitudinal two-dimensional echocardiogram with explanatory diagram. A cardiac catheter is visualized passing a membranous ventricular septal defect from the right ventricle to the left ventricle.

Ao = aorta, PA = pulmonary artery, RV = right ventricle, LV = left ventricle, cath = catheter.

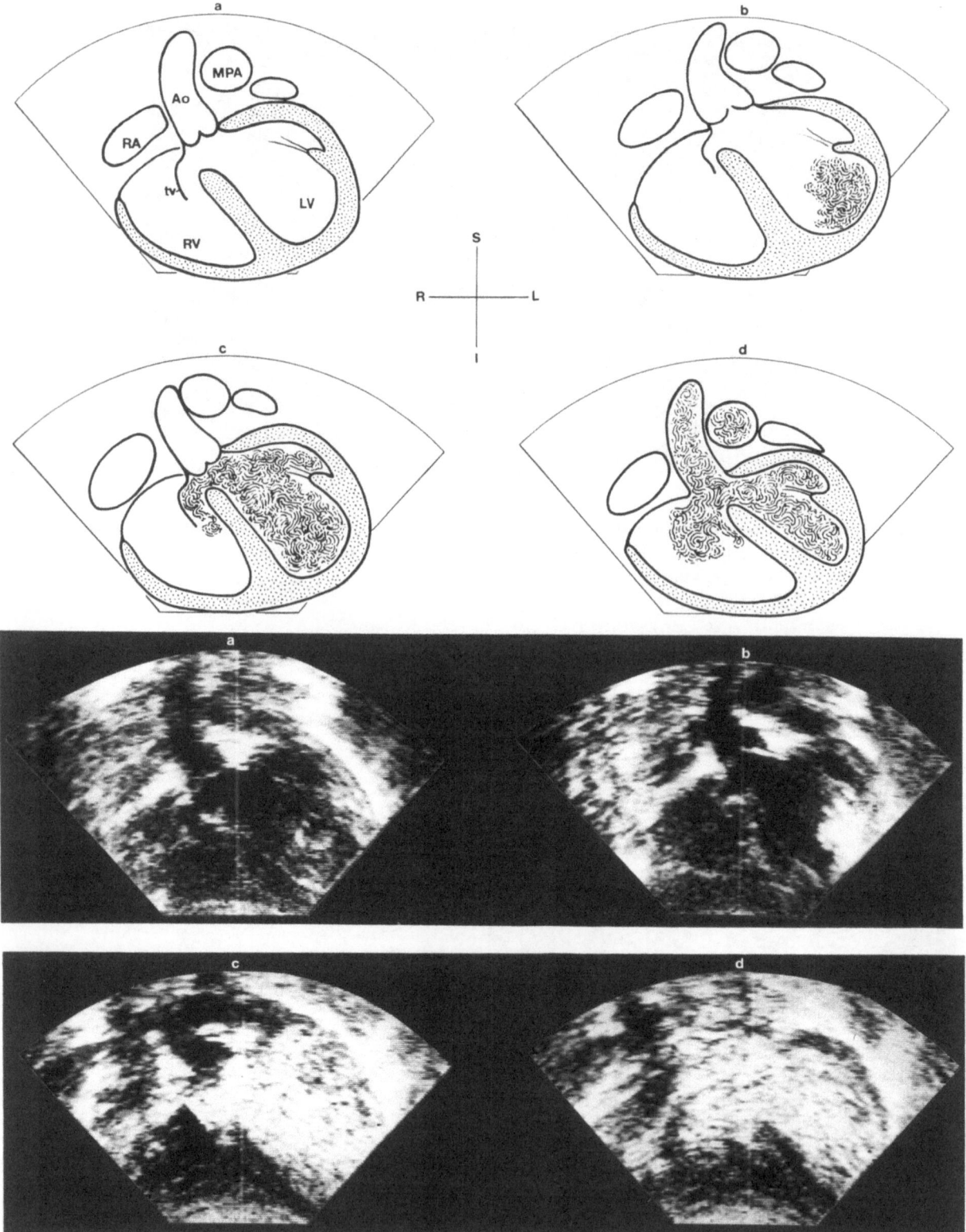

Figure 2.5. Subcostal longitudinal two-dimensional echocardiograms with diagrams of a left ventricular echocontrast study in the same patient with the membranous ventricular septal defect as in Figure 2.4. The contrast appears first in the apex of the left ventricle (b). Immediately afterwards (c) the whole left ventricle is filled with contrast and through the ventricular septal defect there is already some contrast against the septal tricuspid leaflet. Finally the right ventricle is filled with contrast (d) as the result of a large L-R shunt.

RA = right atrium, Ao = aorta, MPA = main pulmonary artery, tv = tricuspid valve, RV = right ventricle, LV = left ventricle.

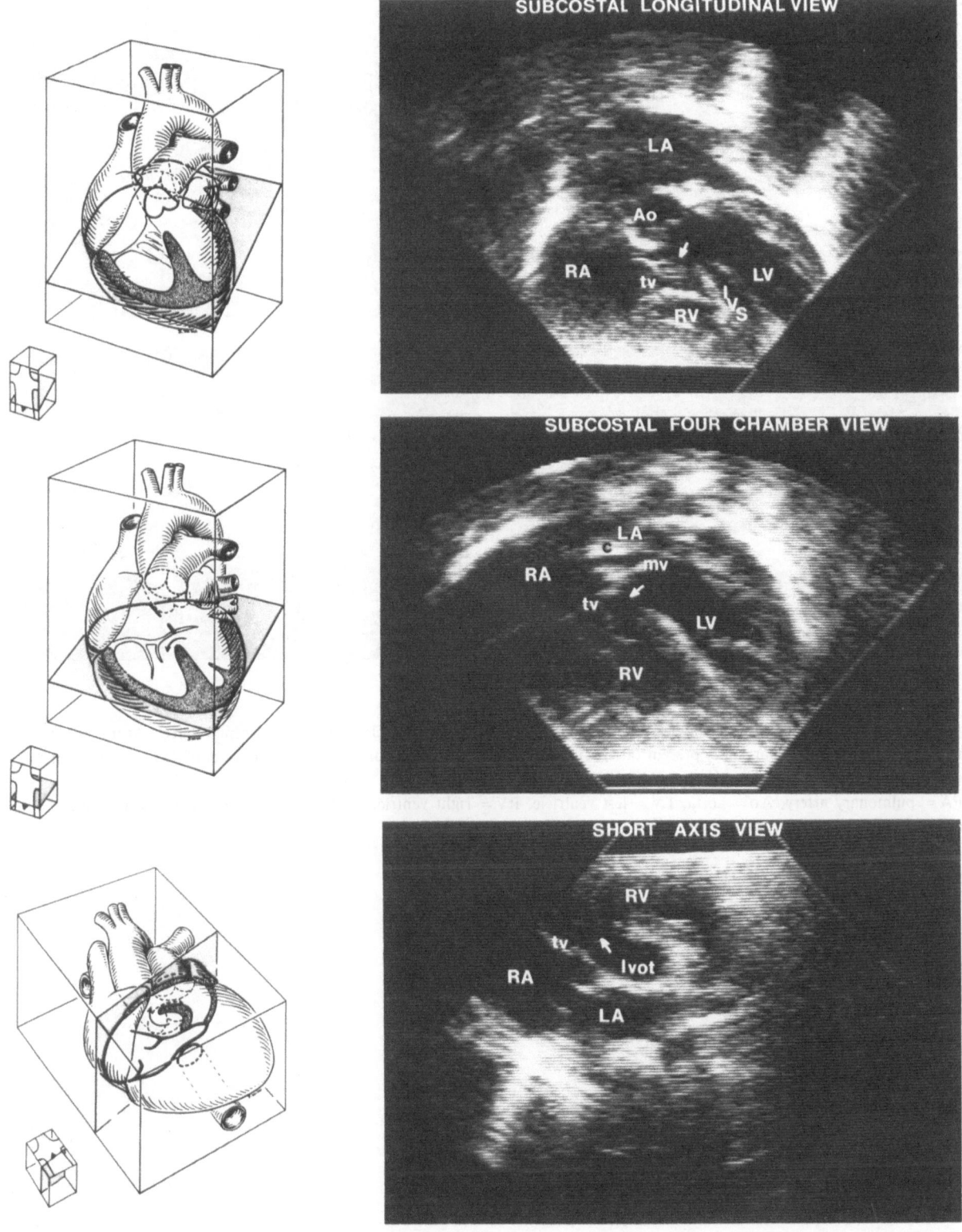

Figure 2.6. Two-dimensional echocardiograms exhibiting a perimembranous inlet ventricular septal defect. Arrows indicate the site of the septal deficiency.

LA = left atrium, Ao = aorta, RA = right atrium, tv = tricuspid valve, RV = right ventricle, IVS = interventricular septum, LV = left ventricle, c = catheter, mv = mitral valve, lvot = left ventricular outflow tract.

32

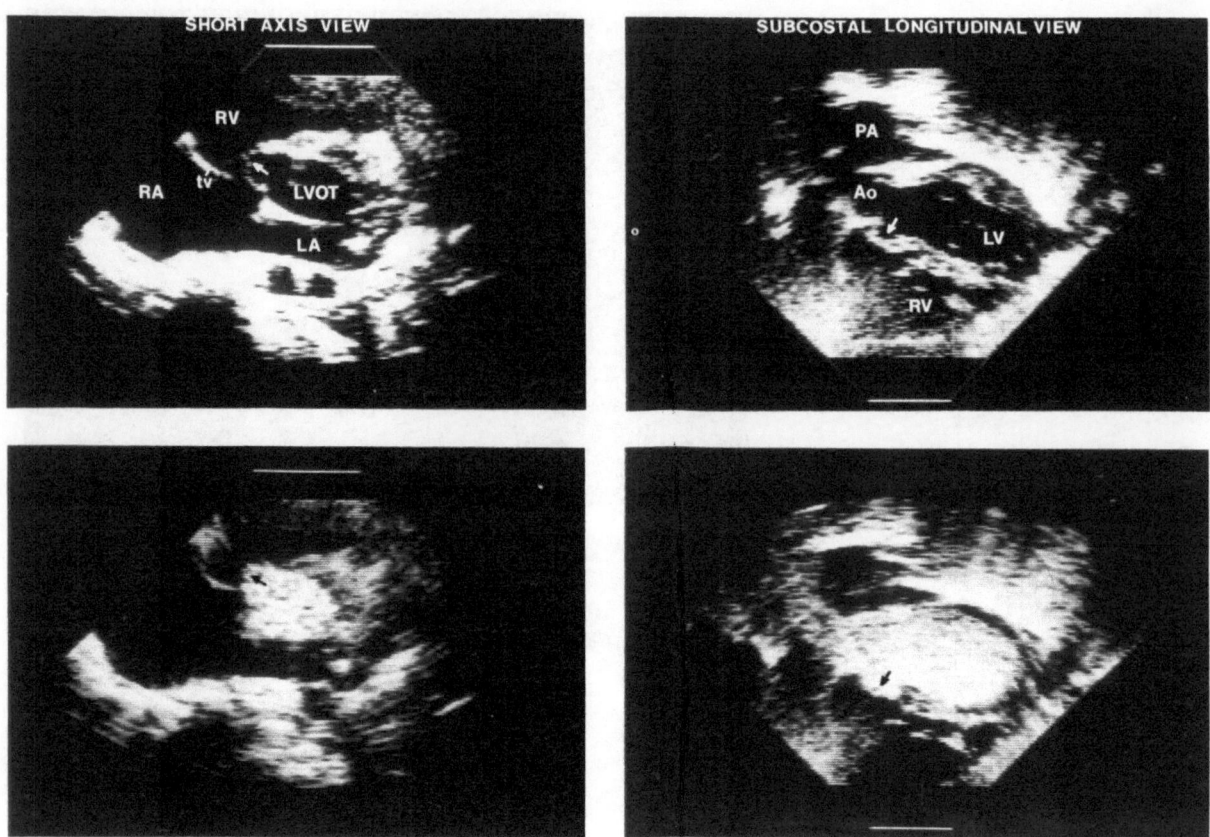

Figure 2.7. Two-dimensional echocardiograms of a patient with a spontaneously closed ventricular septal defect. At the site of the membranous septum an aneurysm is present (arrows). After injection of echocontrast into the left ventricle (lower panels) the aneurysm is filled but a L-R shunt is absent.

PA = pulmonary artery, Ao = aorta, LV = left ventricle, RV = right ventricle, RA = right atrium, LA = left atrium, tv = tricuspid valve, LVOT = left ventricular outflow tract.

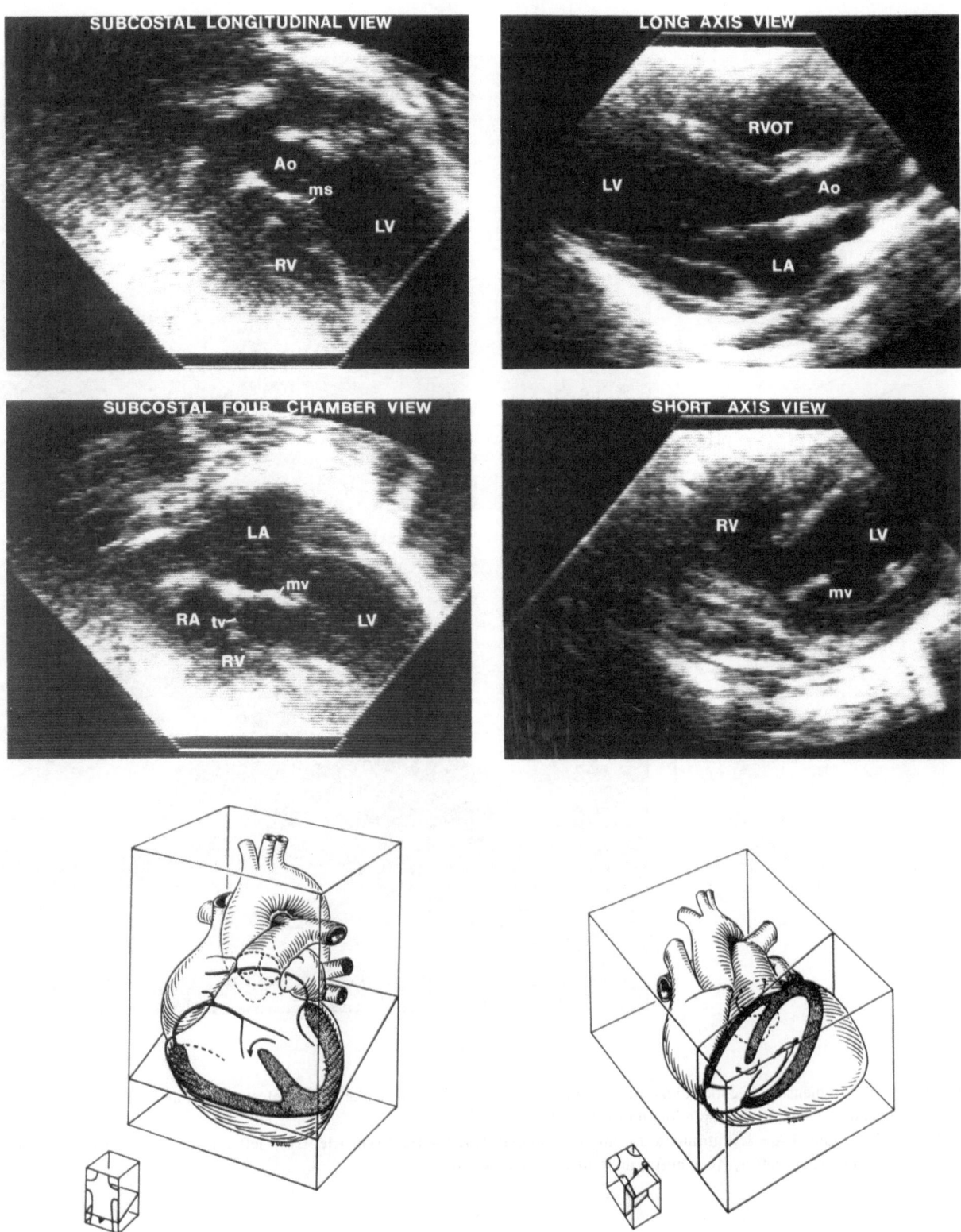

Figure 2.8. Two-dimensional echocardiograms of a patient with a large muscular inlet ventricular septal defect.

Ao = aorta, ms = membranous septum, RV = right ventricle, LV = left ventricle, RVOT = right ventricular outflow tract, LA = left atrium, RA = right atrium, tv = tricuspid valve, mv = mitral valve.

34

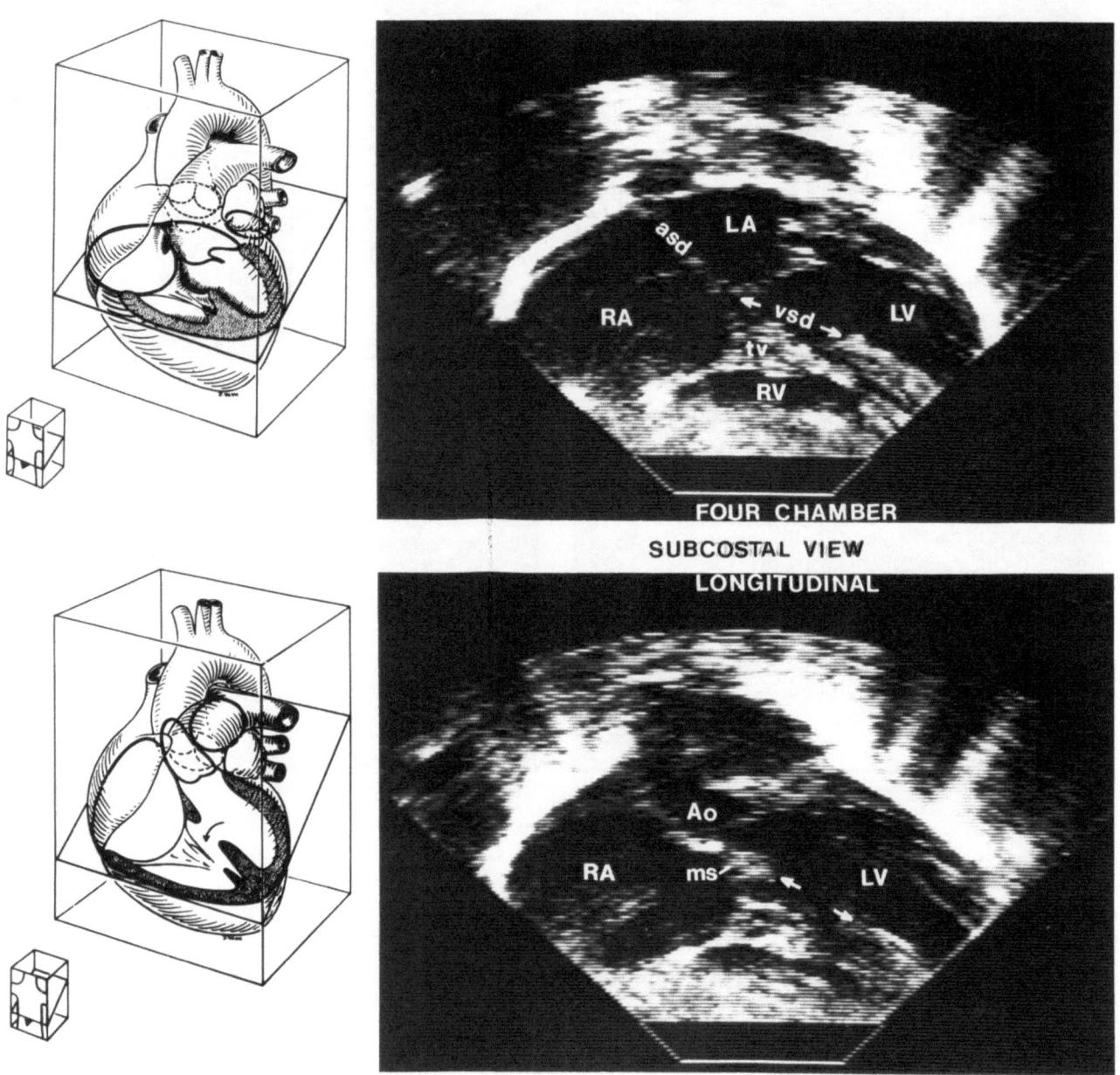

Figure 2.9. Two-dimensional echocardiograms showing a large muscular ventricular septal defect of inlet and trabecular septum. Arrows indicate the superior and inferior rim of the defect.

RA = right atrium, RA = left atrium, asd = atrial septal defect, RV = right ventricle, LV = left ventricle, tv = tricuspid valve, vsd = ventricular septal defect, Ao = aorta, ms = membranous septum.

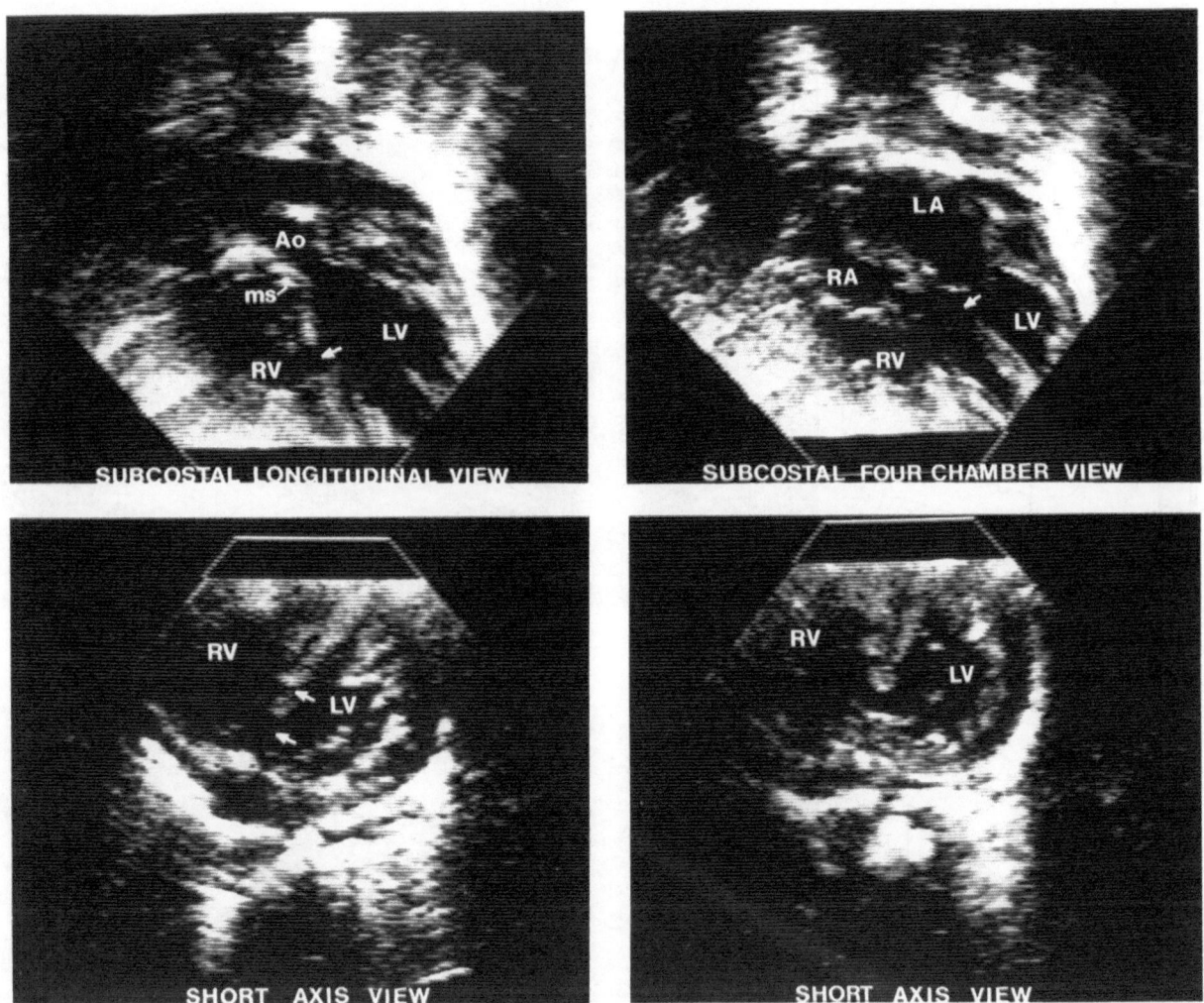

Figure 2.10. Two-dimensional echocardiograms of a patient with two defects in the muscular inlet septum. Arrows indicate the site of the septal deficiencies.

Ao = aorta, ms = membranous septum, RV = right ventricle, LV = left ventricle, RA = right atrium, LA = left atrium.

36

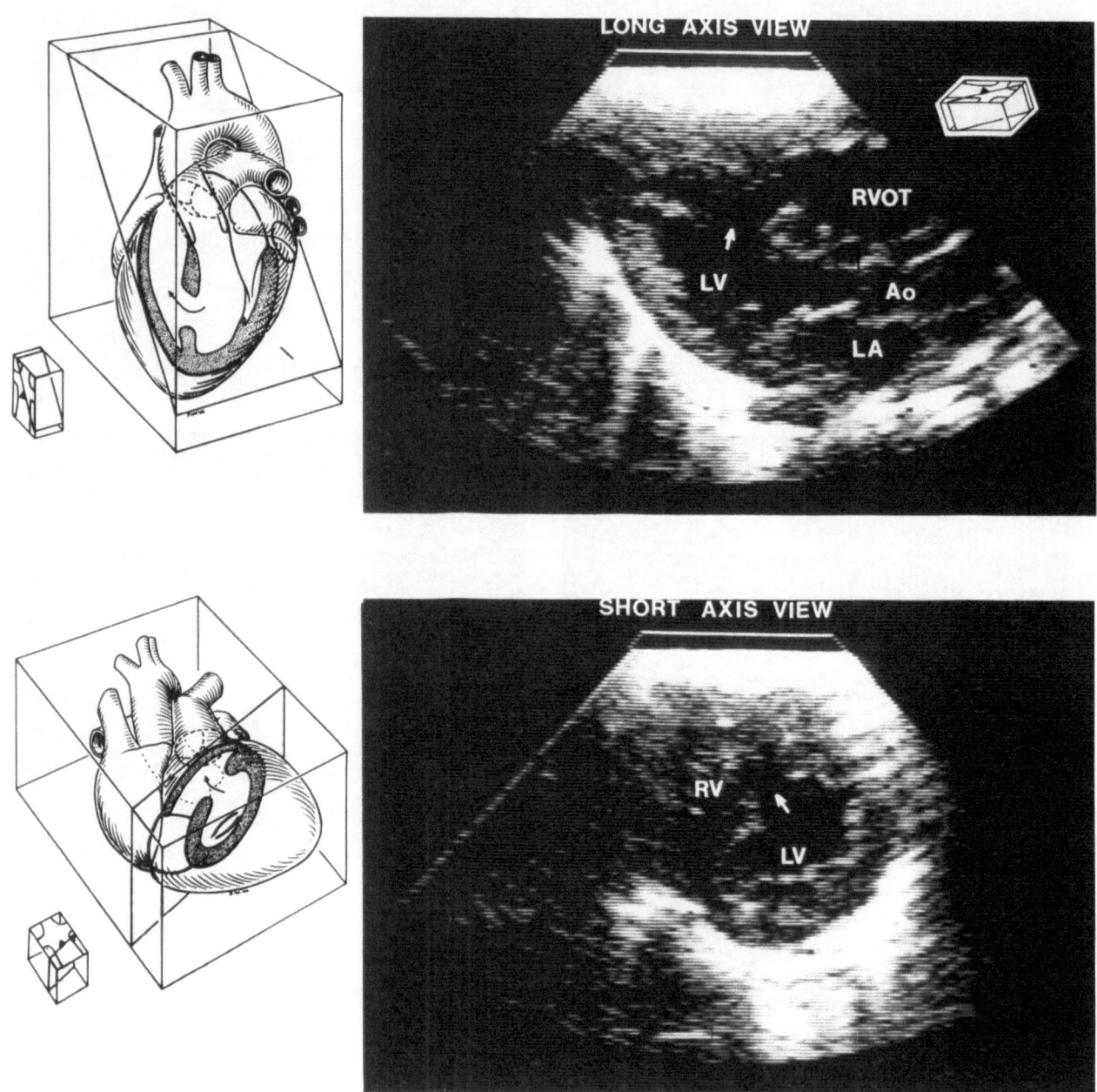

Figure 2.11. Two-dimensional echocardiograms of a patient with a defect in the trabecular part of the interventricular septum. Arrows indicate the site of the septal deficiency.

   LV = left ventricle, RVOT = right ventricular outflow tract, LA = left atrium, Ao = aorta, RV = right ventricle.

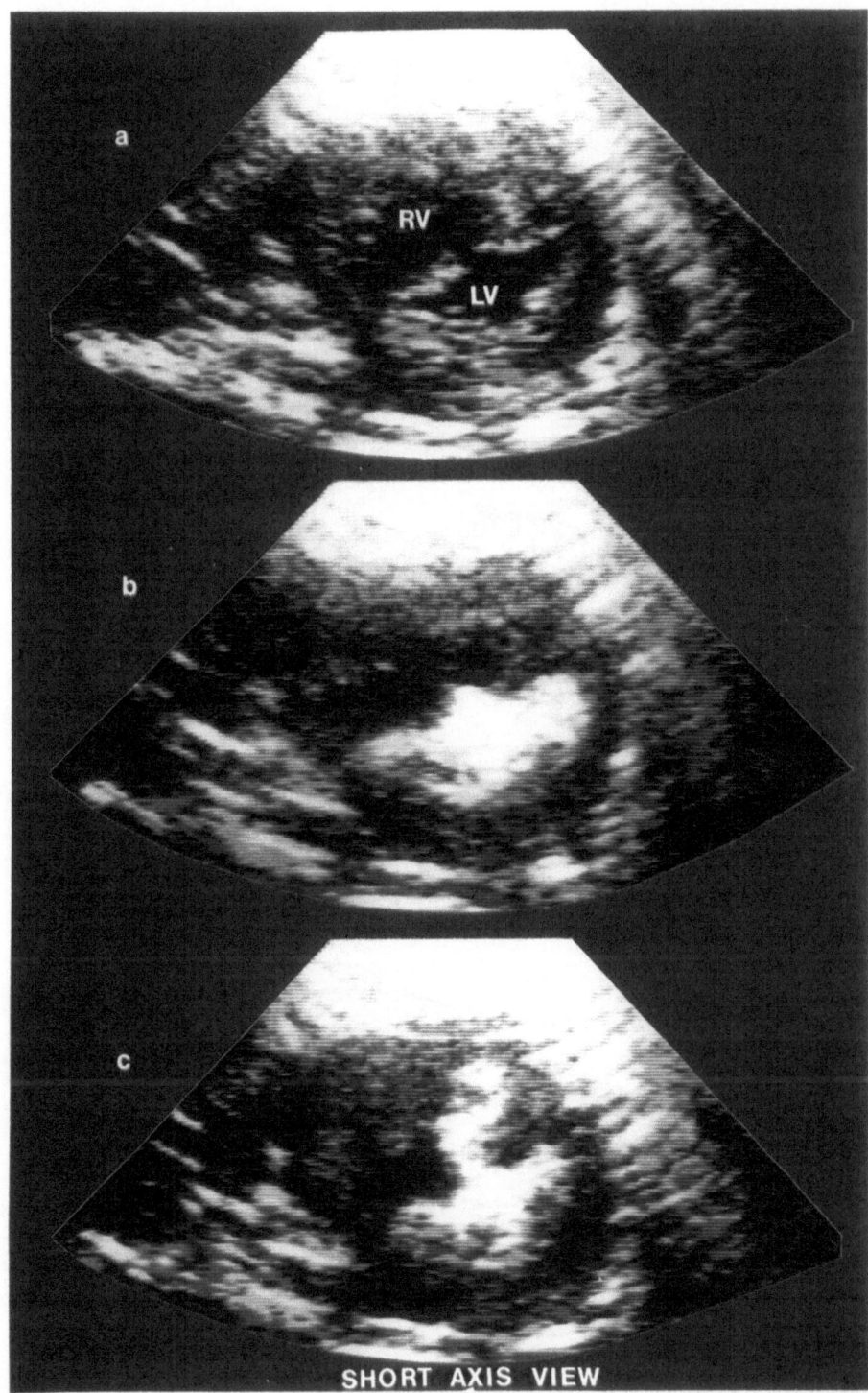

Figure 2.12. Two-dimensional echocardiograms showing a left ventricular echocontrast injection in a patient with trabecular ventricular septal defect.

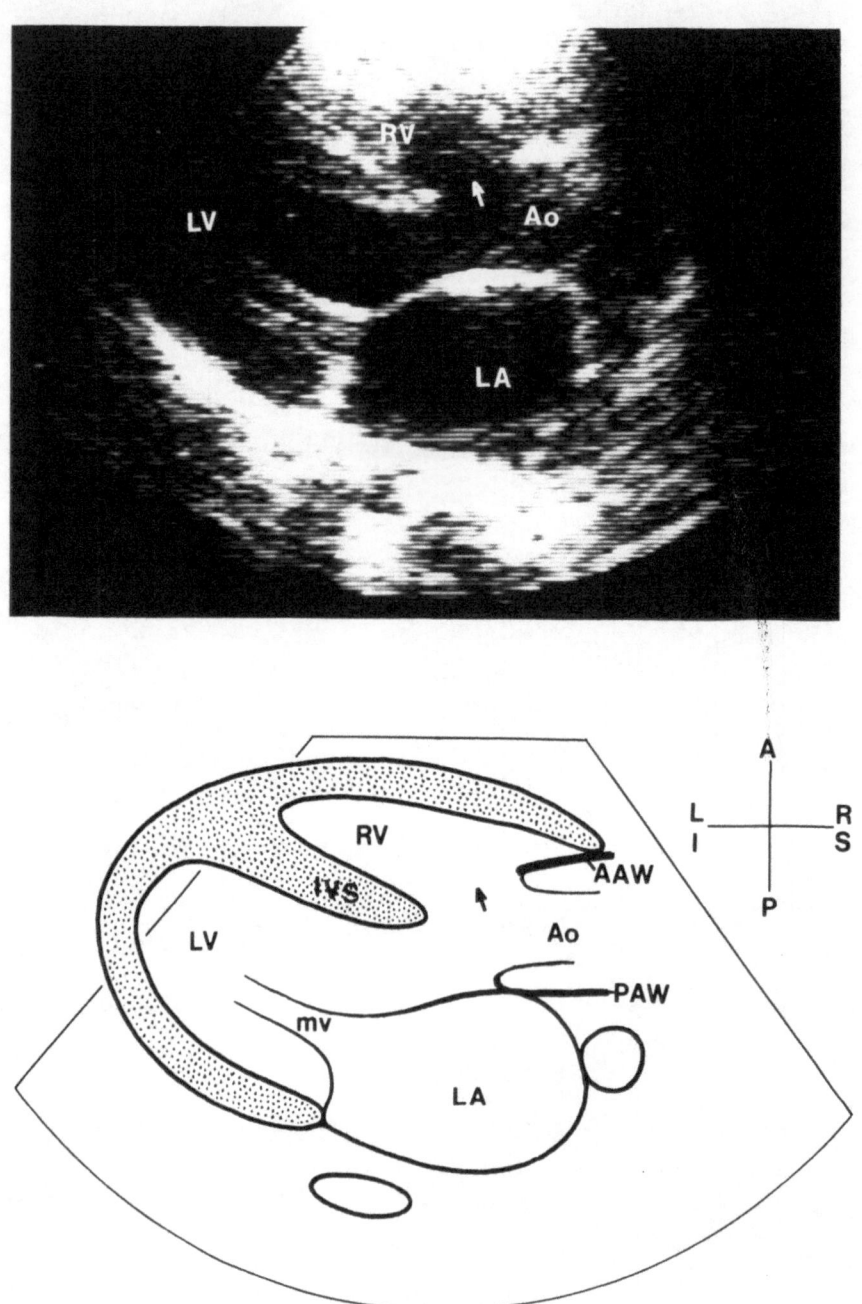

Figure 2.13. Parasternal long axis two-dimensional echocardiogram of a patient with a Fallot-like ventricular septal defect. The arrow indicates the site of the subaortic septal deficiency.

RV = right ventricle, LV = left ventricle, LA = left atrium, Ao = aorta, AAW = anterior aortic wall, PAW = posterior aortic wall, IVS = interventricular septum, mv = mitral valve.

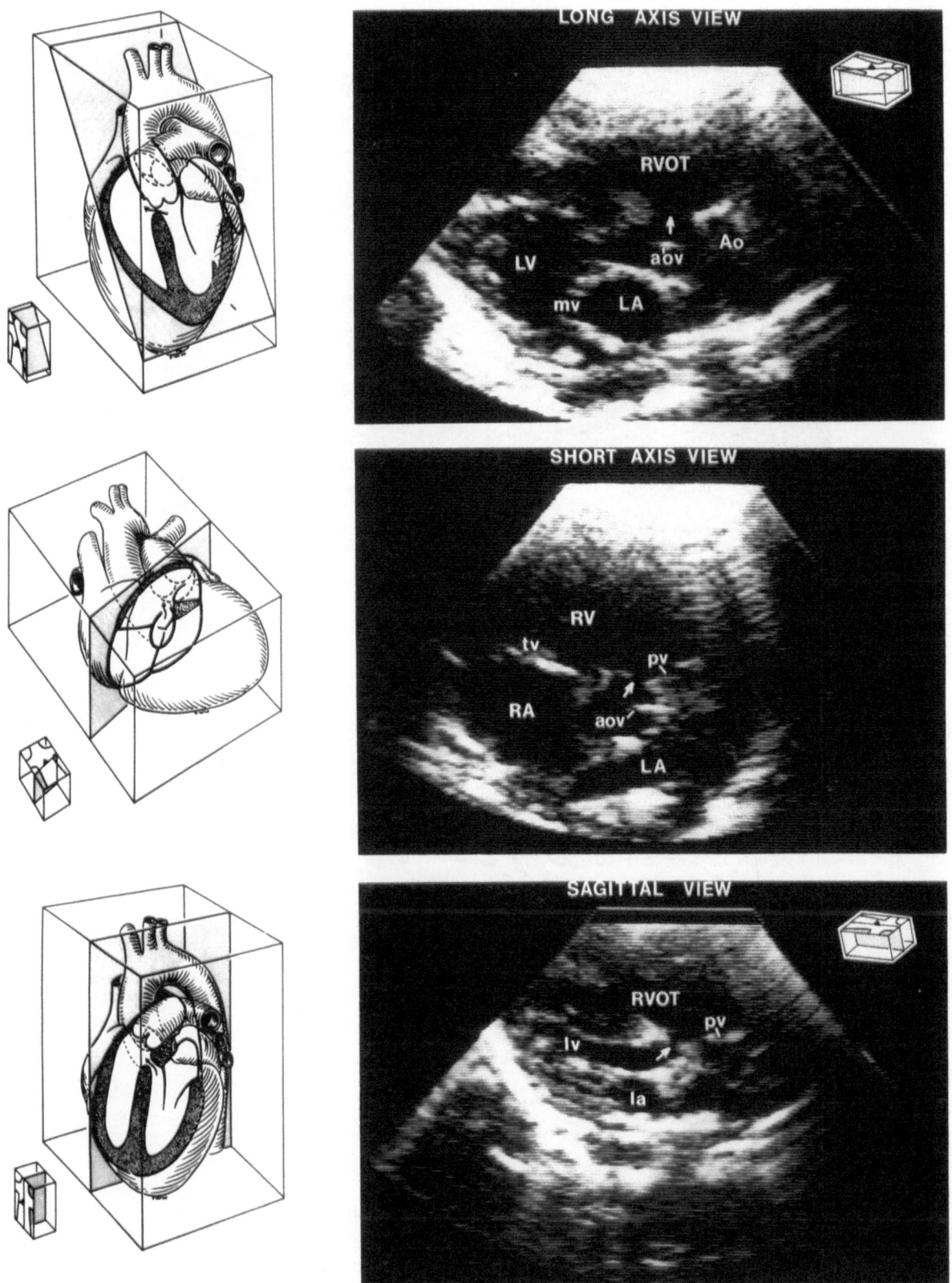

Figure 2.14. Parasternal two-dimensional echocardiograms showing a subarterial outlet ventricular septal defect. The site of the septal deficiency is indicated by an arrow.

RVOT = right ventricular outflow tract, LV, lv = left ventricle, Ao = aorta, aov = aortic valve, LA, la = left atrium, mv = mitral valve, RV = right ventricle, RA = right atrium, tv = tricuspid valve, pv = pulmonary valve.

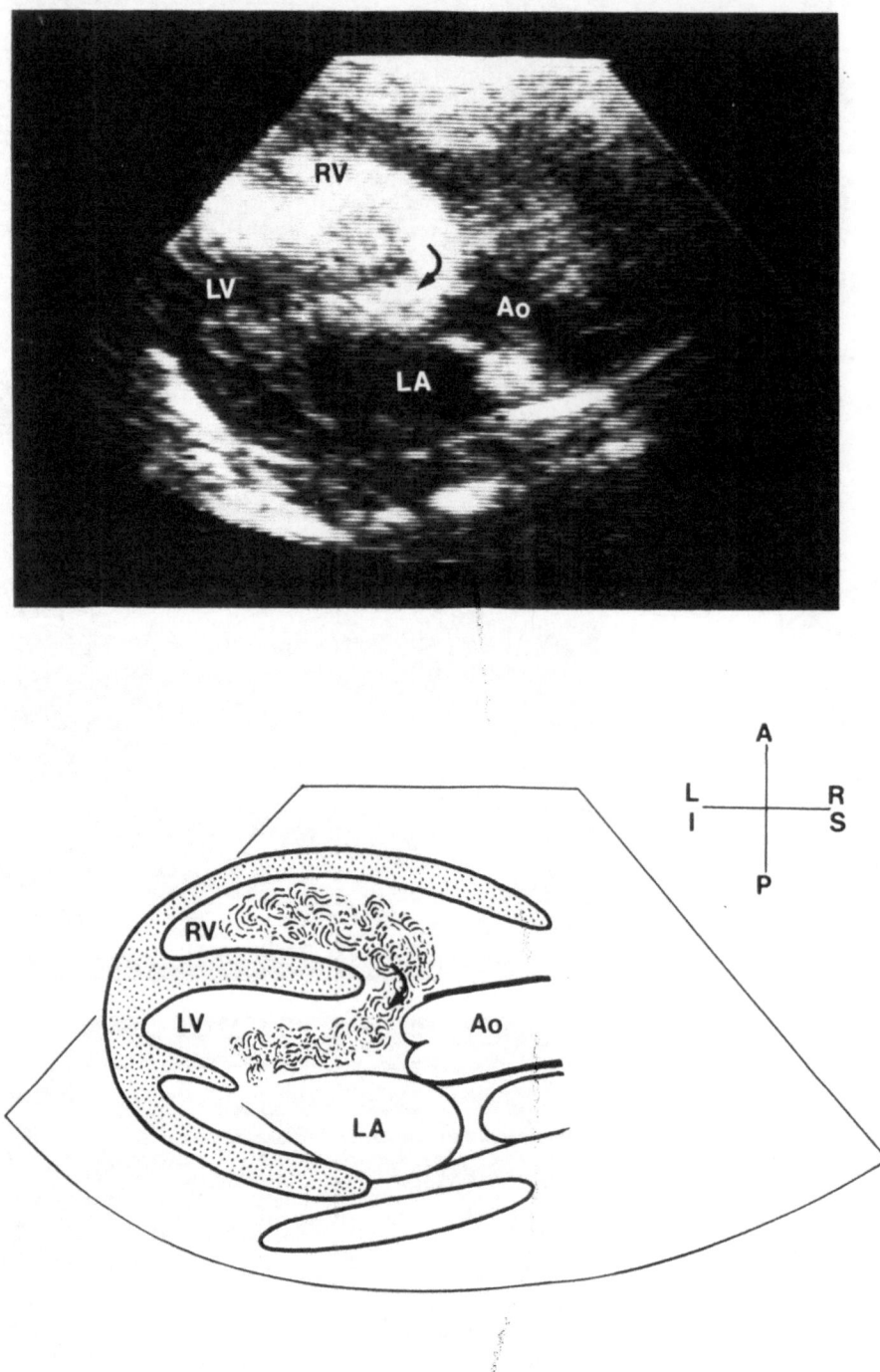

Figure 2.15. Parasternal long axis two-dimensional echocardiogram of the same patient as in Figure 2.14. After a venous echocontrast injection the R-L shunt is visualized.

3. ATRIAL SEPTUM, ATRIAL SEPTAL DEFECT AND ANOMALOUS PULMONARY VENOUS DRAINAGE

Isolated atrial septal defect is seldom diagnosed in the early months of life. The compliance of the right ventricle slowly increases above that of the left ventricle. Consequently, the L-R atrial shunt gradually develops. Furthermore, the L-R shunt in atrial septal defect rarely causes clinical symptoms. The patient is commonly referred to the pediatric cardiologist for analysis of a cardiac murmur. An ejection murmur over the pulmonary area with typical fixed splitting of the second sound with a loud pulmonary component is usually the first sign of an atrial septal defect with a significant L-R shunt. In these cases the chest X-ray reveals increased pulmonary vascular markings and cardiomegaly. The cardiomegaly is mainly due to the dilated right ventricle which is readily observed by echocardiography. The absence of evidence of pulmonary hypertension on the pulmonary valve M-mode echocardiogram and the possible presence of paradoxical septal motion indicate that volume overload is the only cause of the right ventricular dilatation. Two-dimensional echocardiography reveals normal attachment of the tricuspid valve without a significant prolapse. The atrial septal defect is best visualized directly in the subcostal four chamber view because in this cross-section the ultrasound beam has a more perpendicular relation with the atrial septum compared with other views. The apical four chamber view (2) and the parasternal short axis view, at the level of the great arteries (3), may also be used but ultrasound coming from these windows tends to pass parallel to the atrial septum. Therefore, central septal 'dropouts' easily occur, particularly when the overall resolution is inadequate or the gainsettings are not properly adjusted.

Figure 3.1 and 3.2 show subcostal four chamber views of a patient with a large central atrial septal defect. The diameter of the defect in this case is nearly 1 cm. The left and right inferior pulmonary veins clearly enter the left atrium. As in ventricular septal defects the edges of an atrial septal defect can show a T-artefact (Figure 3.3). A large dorsal atrial septal defect is displayed in Figure 3.4. The ventral part of the atrial septum only is present (4). The ventrally situated atrial septal defect is described with the atrioventricular septal defects (chapter 4). Figure 3.5 shows a central atrial septal defect visualized in the parasternal short axis view.

In atrial septal defect peripheral venous echocontrast studies can confirm the diagnosis by visualizing a R-L atrial shunt or a negative contrast effect (5, 6). In our experience with children physical examination, chest X-ray and two-dimensional echocardiography without echocontrast studies will accurately detect a haemodynamically important atrial septal defect.

In transposition of the great arteries with intact ventricular septum an interatrial communication is imperative to establish an adequate bi-directional shunt. Hence, balloon atrial septostomy is necessary shortly after birth. This procedure can be carried out under two-dimensional echocardiographic control (Figure 3.6). The result can be estimated by direct visualization of the opening in the atrial septum. Real-time imaging reveals the flapping tissue of the ruptured membrane of the foramen ovale in case of adequate atrial septostomy. Furthermore, echocontrast injections into the atria may give an impression in some degree of the magnitude of the bi-directional shunt.

Partial abnormal drainage of the pulmonary veins can be identified or excluded by echocontrast studies during cardiac catheterization. When the tip of the cardiac catheter is manipulated into the suspected abnormal pulmonary vein injection of echocontrast will reveal whether contrast enters the heart to the right or to the left of the atrial septum.

Direct visualisation of the site of partial abnormal drainage of the pulmonary veins into the superior vena cava or right atrium has, as far as the authors know, not been described. As an isolated lesion this anomaly should be suspected if there is echocardiographic evidence of right ventricle volume overload with intact interatrial septum. In total anomalous pulmonary venous drainage filling of the left atrium depends entirely on the R-L shunt through a foramen ovale or an atrial septal defect. The subcostal or apical four chamber view will fail to visualize the normal entry of the pulmonary veins. Echocontrast injections into a peripheral vein will demonstrate the R-L atrial shunt. The combination of these two observations are very suspect for the diagnosis total anomalous pulmonary venous drainage. Differentiation between total anomalous pulmonary venous drainage and pulmonary hypoperfusion in persistent foetal circulation syndrome may be difficult. In the latter the pulmonary veins are collapsed and therefore may be difficult to recognize. The two-dimensional echocardiographic findings of an additional space, superior and posterior or lateral to the left atrium, into which the pulmonary veins enter is in favour of total anomalous pulmonary drainage. This is the common pulmonary vein (Figure 3.7). Assessment of the abnormal site of drainage of the pulmonary veins in total anomalous pulmonary venous drainage should be possible (7, 8). In this respect Smallhorn and associates (8) stress the importance of the suprasternal approach. The two-dimensional echocardiograms of a patient with a supracardiac type of total anomalous pulmonary venous drainage is exhibited in Figure 3.8. Multiple parasternal views and a subcostal frontal view portray the abnormal course of the pulmonary venous channel to the superior vena cava.

Total anomalous pulmonary venous drainage must be distinguished from cor triatriatum sinister. In the latter condition the pulmonary veins drain directly into the dorsal region of the left atrium. The ventral region of the left atrium communicates with the left ventricle and is separated from the dorsal part by an intra-atrial membrane (Fig. 3.9). Through one or more small apertures in this membrane the pulmonary venous blood reaches the ventral part of the left atrium. If these openings cannot be visualized the dorsal part of the left atrium may be confused with the common pulmonary vein into which the pulmonary veins enter in total anomalous pulmonary venous drainage. The absence of a drainage vessel and the insertion of the intra-atrial membrane into the middle of the interatrial septum are indicative of cor triatriatum sinister.

In complex structural heart defects interatrial communication may be imperative to maintain haemodynamic stability. For instance, an interatrial communication is an integral part of tricuspid atresia. It is the only means of exit of venous blood from the right atrium. In hypoplastic left heart syndrome this communication allows the essential L-R atrial shunt. A pressure gradient across the atrial septum is only present when the interatrial defect is small. In large atrial septal defects there is no atrial pressure difference. If there is a pressure gradient the atrial septum may be convex to the atrium with the lowest pressure. Hence, bulging of the atrial septum may be a rough indication of the pressure relationship between the two atria and may be suggestive for an obstructive lesion in one or other side of the heart. The curvature of the atrial septum is maximal during diastole when the pressure gradient is maximal. An additional circumscript protuberance of the atrial septum may be identified at the site of the foramen ovale. If marked this is said to be an 'aneurysm' of the membranous fossa ovalis (9). Severe bulging of the atrial septum into the left atrium suggests a severe obstruction on the right side of the heart such as tricuspid, or pulmonary stenosis or atresia, or extreme high pulmonary vascular resistance e.g. in persistent foetal circulation syndrome (Figure 3.10 and Figure 3.11). Echocontrast injections into a peripheral vein may show the concomitant R-L atrial shunt and possibly delayed emptying of the right atrium. Severe bulging of the atrial septum into the right atrium suggests a left-sided obstructive lesion as shown in Figure 3.12. However, one should realize that a convexity of the atrial septum to the right may also be caused by severe volume overload of the left atrium (Figure 3.13).

References

1. Bierman FZ, Williams RG: Subxiphoid two-dimensional imaging of the interatrial septum in infants and neonates with congenital heart disease. Circulation 60:80 – 90, 1979.

2. Silverman NH, Schiller NB: Apex echocardiography. A two-dimensional technique for evaluating congenital heart disease. Circulation 57:503 – 511, 1978.

3. Dillon JC, Weyman AE, Feigenbaum H, Eggleton RC, Johnston K: Cross-sectional echocardiographic examination of the interatrial septum. Circulation 55:115 – 120, 1977.

4. Nasser FN, Tajik AJ, Seward JB, Hagler DJ: Diagnosis of sinus venosus atrial septal defect by two-dimensional echocardiography. Mayo Clin Proc 56:568 – 572, 1981.

5. Fraker TD, Harris PJ, Behar VS, Kisslo JA: Detection and exclusion of interatrial shunts by two-dimensional echocardiography and peripheral venous injection. Circulation 59:379 – 384, 1977.

6. Weyman AE, Sam Wann L, Caldwell RL, Hurwitz RA, Dillon JC, Feigenbaum H: Negative contrast echocardiography: a new method for detecting left-to-right shunts. Circulation 59:498 – 505, 1979.

7. Sahn DJ, Allen HD, Lange LW, Goldberg SJ: Cross-sectional echocardiographic diagnosis of the sites of total anomalous pulmonary venous drainage. Circulation 60:1317 – 1325, 1979.

8. Smallhorn JF, Sutherland GR, Tommassini G, Hunter S, Anderson RH, Macartney FJ: Assessment of total anomalous pulmonary venous connection by two-dimensional echocardiography. Br Heart J 46:613 – 623, 1981.

9. Gondi B, Nanda N: Two-dimensional echocardiographic features of atrial septal aneurysms. Circulation 63:452 – 457, 1981.

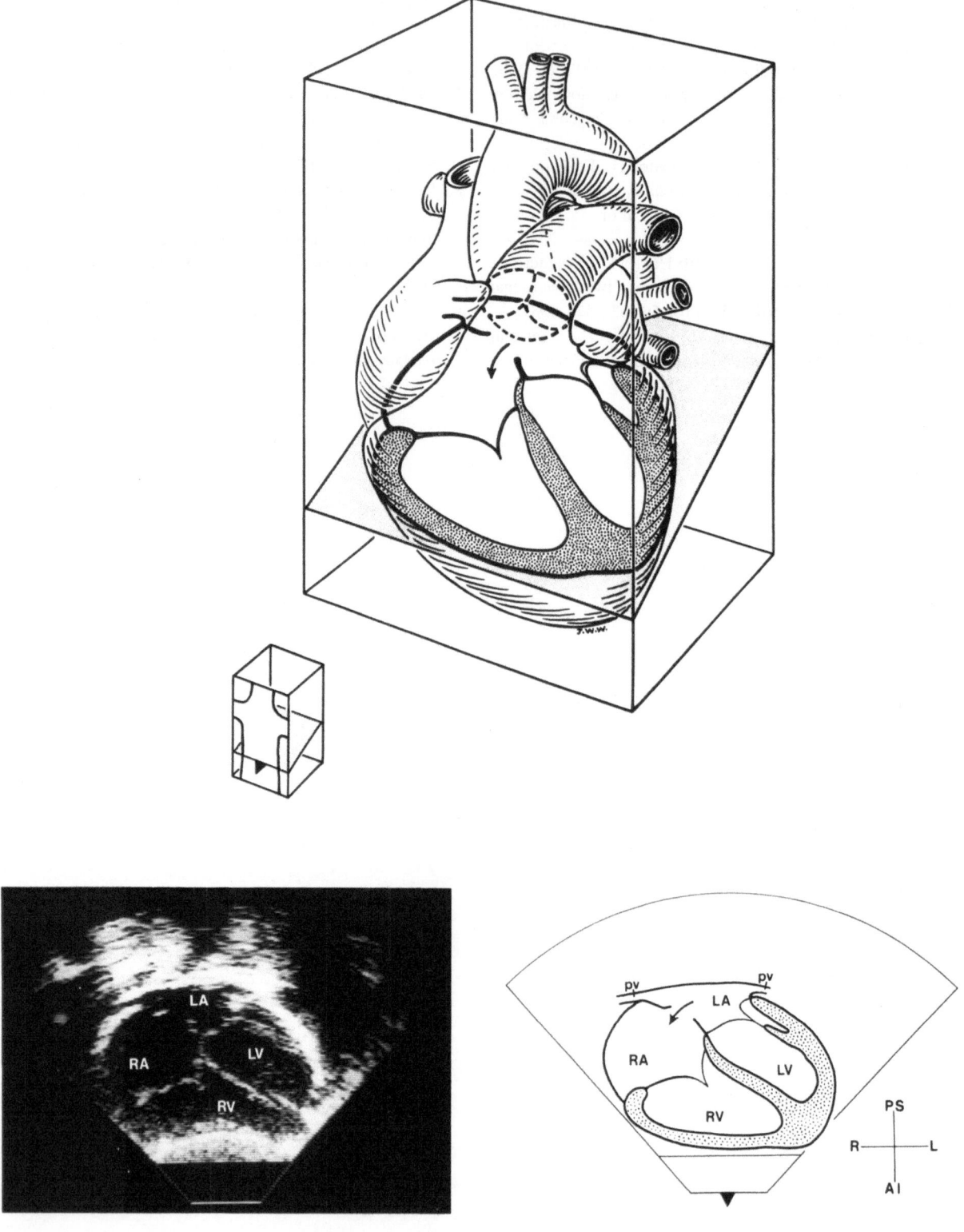

Figure 3.1. Subcostal four chamber two-dimensional echocardiogram of a patient with a secundum (central) atrial septal defect. RA = right atrium, LA = left atrium, pv = pulmonary vein, RV = right ventricle, LV = left ventricle.

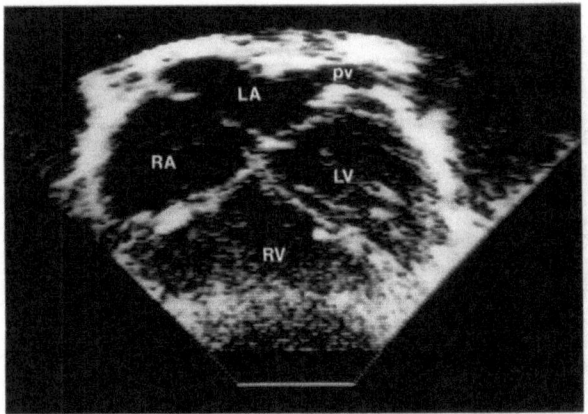

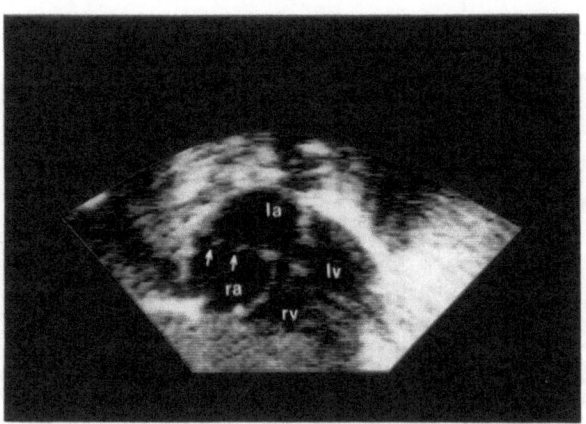

Figure 3.2. Subcostal four chamber view of the same patient as in Figure 3.1. The remaining parts of the interatrial septum are more clearly visualized.

RA = right atrium, LA = left atrium, pv = pulmonary valve, RV = right ventricle, LV = left ventricle.

Figure 3.3. Subcostal four chamber two-dimensional echocardiogram of a patient with a central atrial septal defect. The rims of the defect show a T-artefact (arrows).

ra = right atrium, la = left atrium, rv = right ventricle, lv = left ventricle.

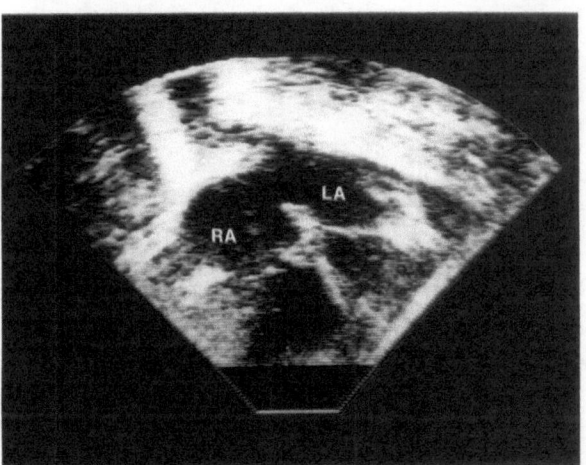

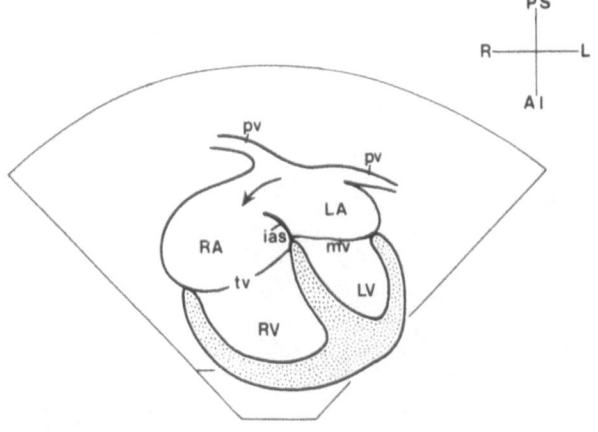

Figure 3.4. Subcostal four chamber two-dimensional echocardiogram of a patient with a dorsal atrial septal defect.

pv = pulmonary vein, RA = right atrium, LA = left atrium, ias = interatrial septum, tv = tricuspid valve, mv = mitral valve, RV = right ventricle, LV = left ventricle.

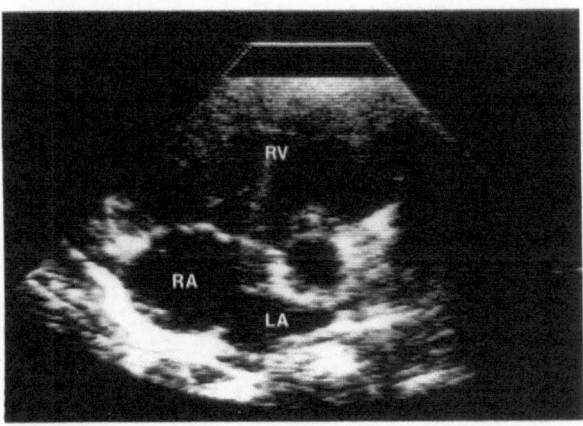

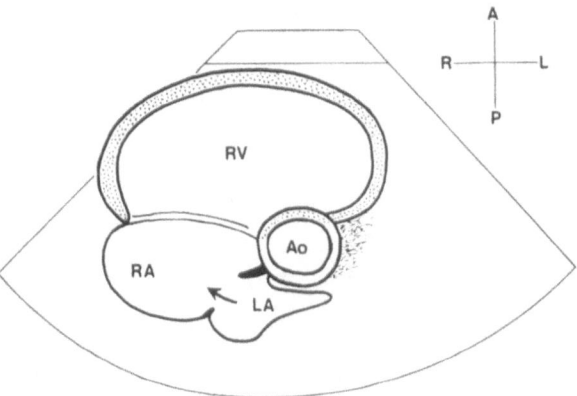

Figure 3.5. Parasternal short axis two-dimensional echocardiogram of a patient with a large secundum (central) atrial septal defect.

RV = *right ventricle*, RA = right atrium, LA = left atrium, Ao = aorta.

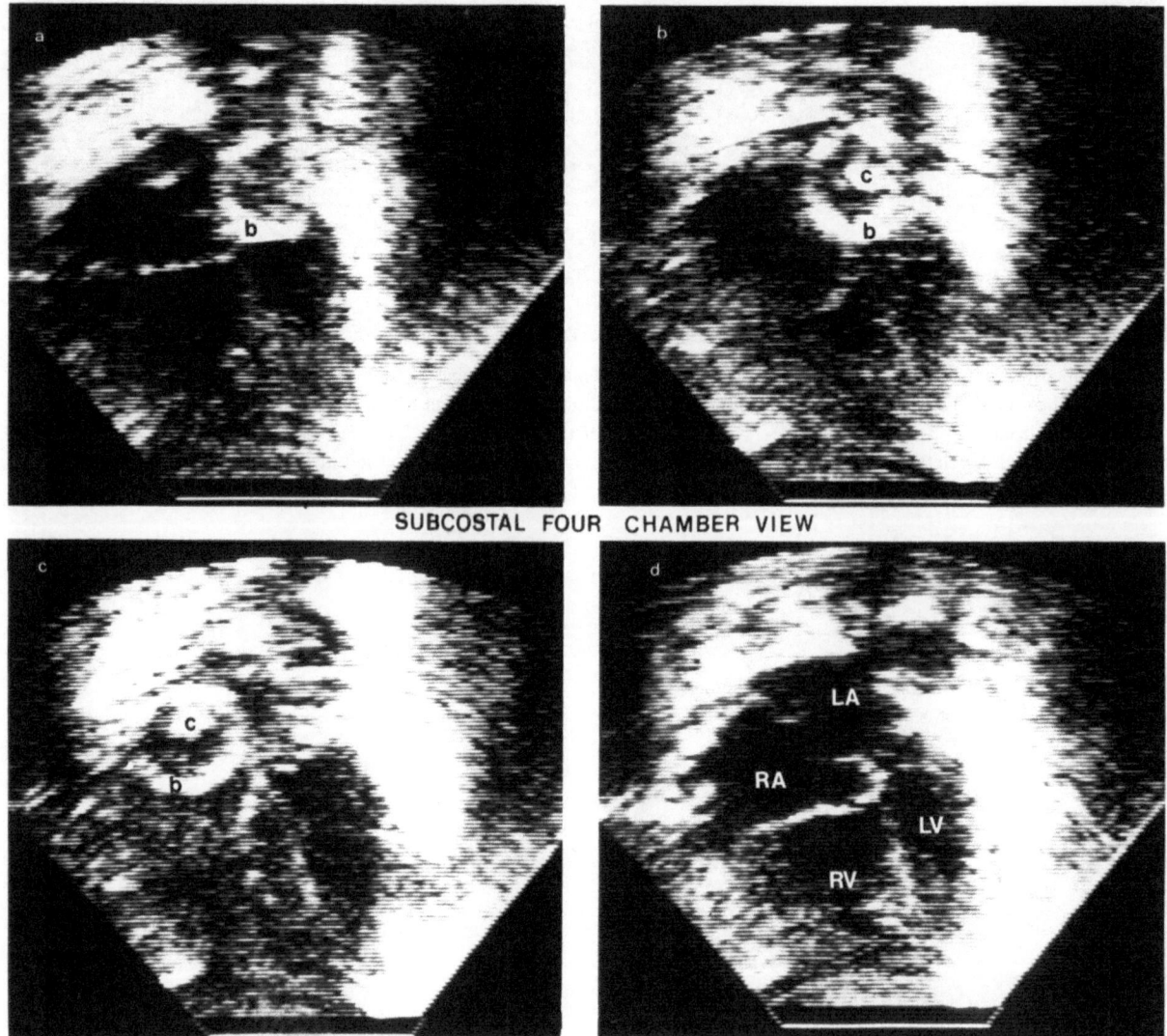

SUBCOSTAL FOUR CHAMBER VIEW

Figure 3.6. Two-dimensional echocardiograms of a patient with transposition of the great arteries. A balloon catheter is introduced into the left atrium through the foramen ovale and the balloon is inflated (a). The catheter is pulled back and the balloon is pressed against the left side of the interatrial septum (b). The balloon has passed the interatrial septum and is visible in the right atrium (c). The balloon is deflated and the catheter removed (d). The result of the procedure can now be assessed.

RA = right atrium, LA = left atrium, RV = right ventricle, LV = left ventricle, b = balloon, c = catheter.

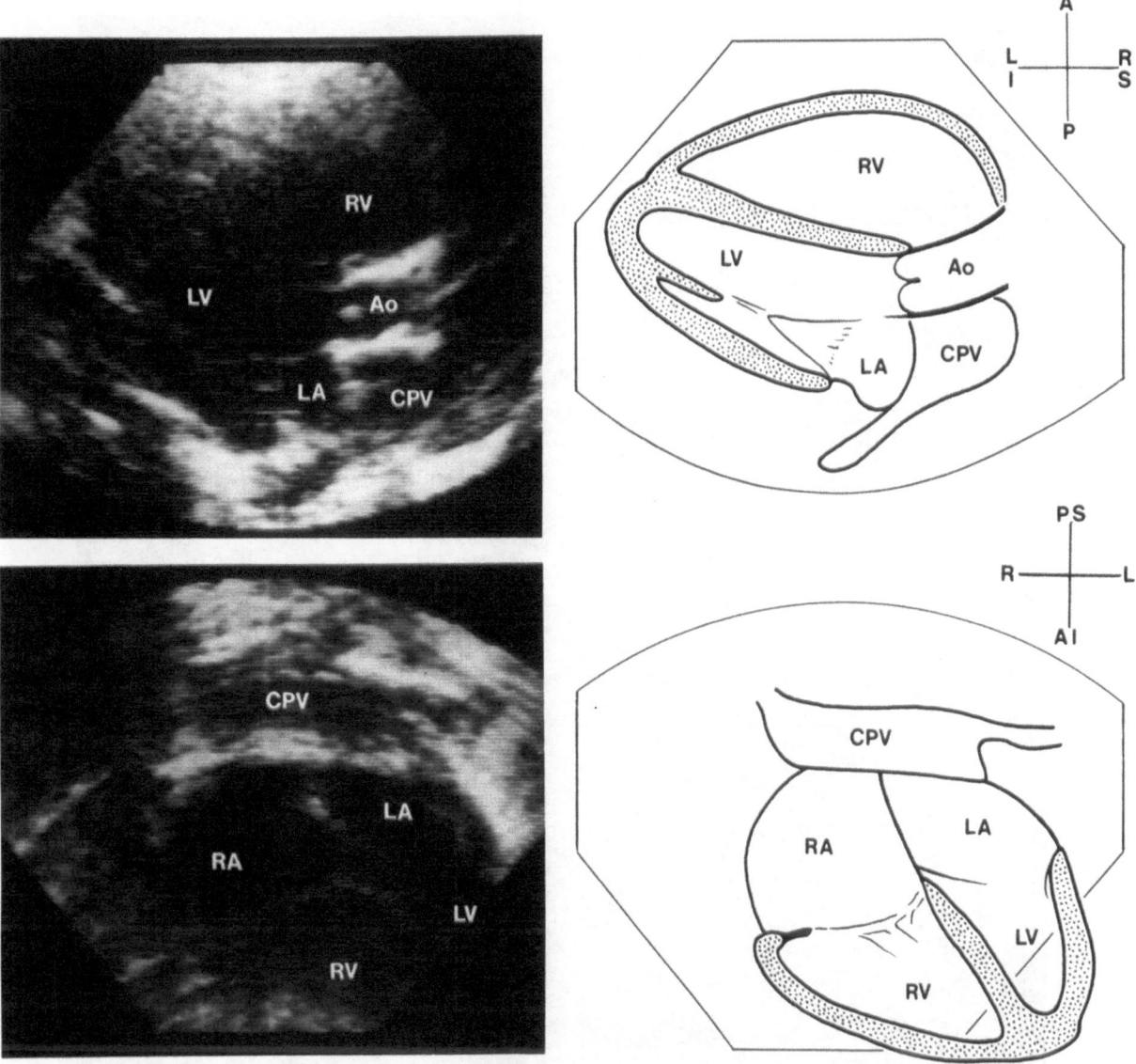

Figure 3.7. Parasternal long axis view (left) and subcostal four chamber view (right) of a patient with total anomalous pulmonary venous return.

CPV = common pulmonary vein, LV = left ventricle, RV = right ventricle, LA = left atrium, RA = right atrium, Ao = aorta.

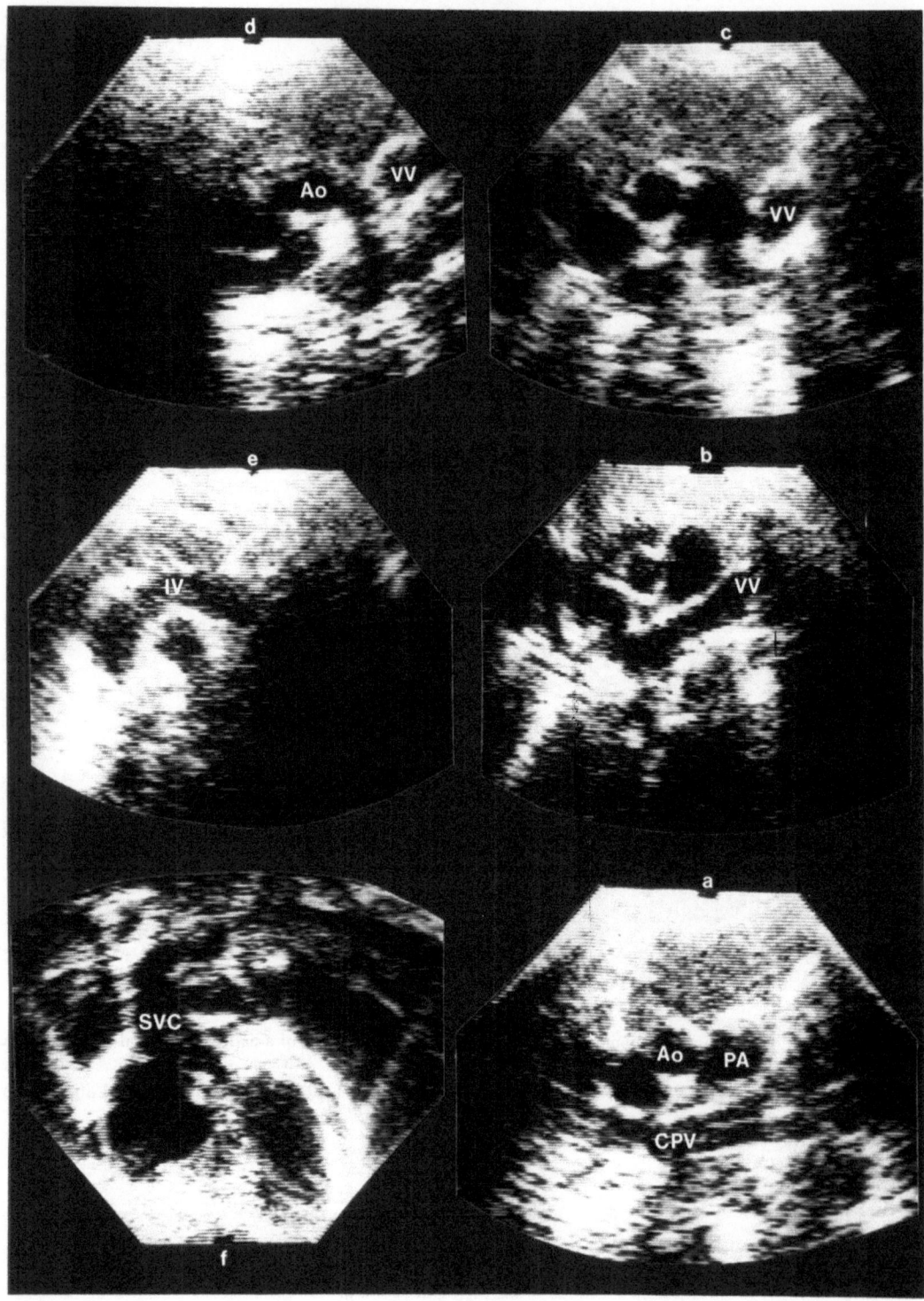

Figure 3.8. For legend see next page.

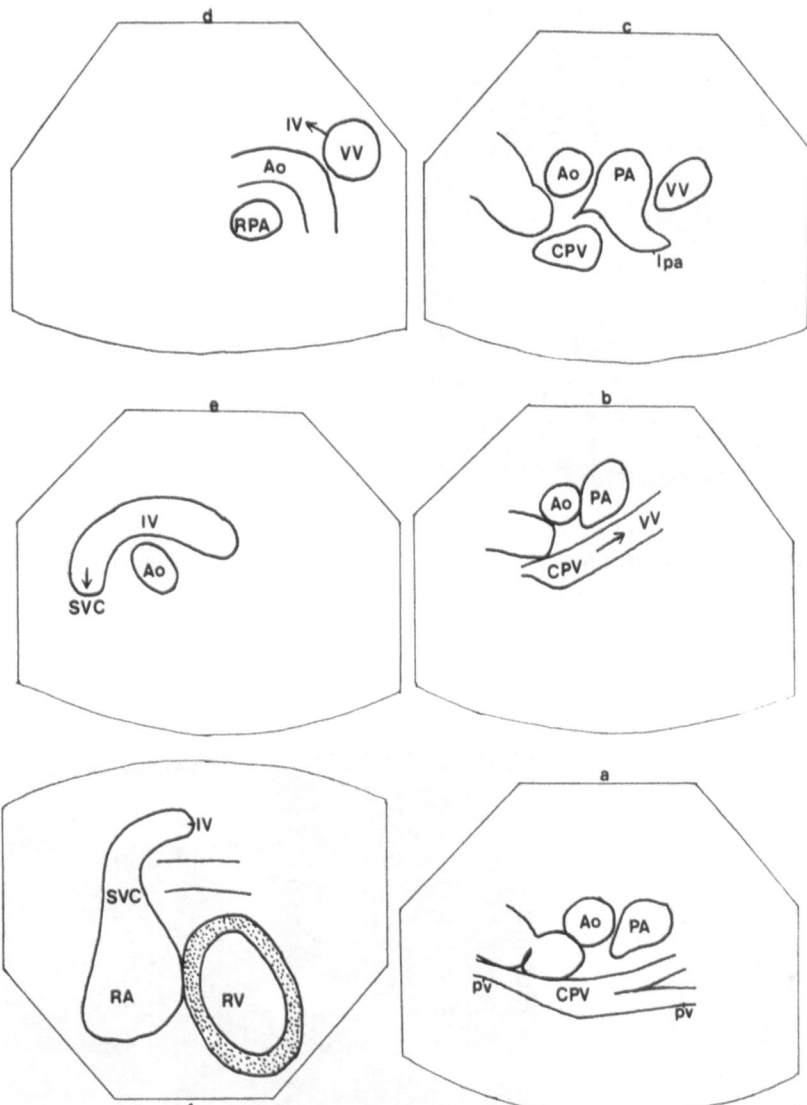

Figure 3.8. Two-dimensional echocardiograms of a patient with a supracardiac type of total anomalous pulmonary venous return. In the short axis view, on the level of the great arteries, the aorta and the pulmonary artery are visualized (a). Behind these vessels the common pulmonary vein is visible receiving the pulmonary veins. While tilting the ultrasonic beam cranially the common pulmonary vein proceeds inferior to the left branch of the pulmonary artery into a left-sided vertical vein (b, c). By moving the transducer superiorly this vertical vein could be followed up to the level of the aortic arch (d). Rotation of the transducer in this position reveals the continuation of the vertical vein to the right into a wide innominate vein superior to the aorta (e). In a subcostal frontal view the entry of the wide innominate vein into the superior caval vein is visualized (f).

pv = pulmonary vein, CPV = common pulmonary vein, Ao = aorta, PA = pulmonary artery, VV = vertical vein, lpa = left pulmonary artery, IV = innominate vein, RPA = right pulmonary artery, SVC = superior vena cava, RA = right atrium, RV = right ventricle.

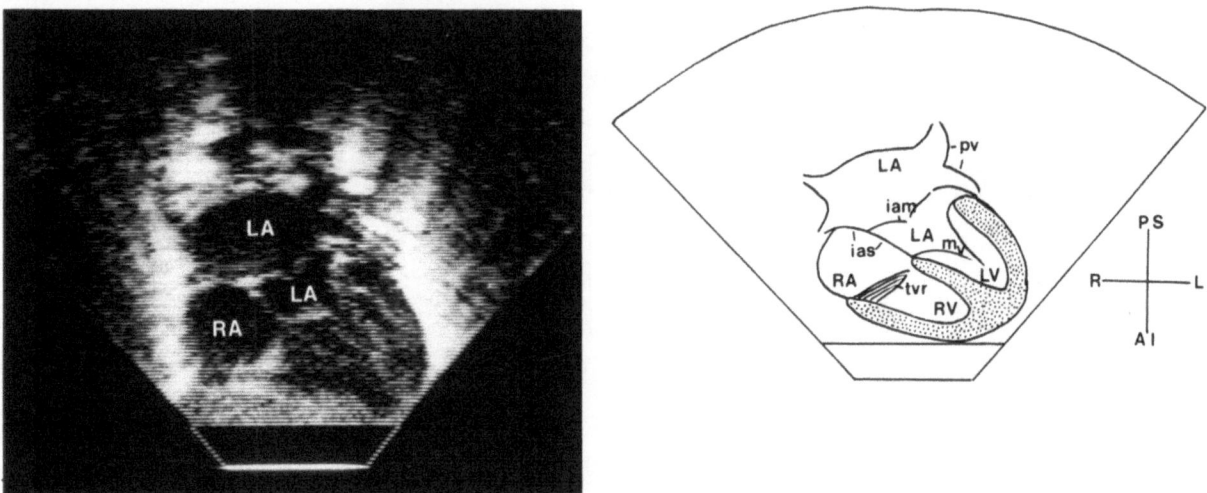

Fig. 3.9. Subcostal four chamber view of a patient with cor triatriatum sinister.
RA = right atrium, RV = right ventricle, LA = left atrium, LV = left ventricle, ias = interatrial septum, iam = intra-atrial membrane, pv = pulmonary valve, mv = mitral valve, tvr = tricuspid valve ring.

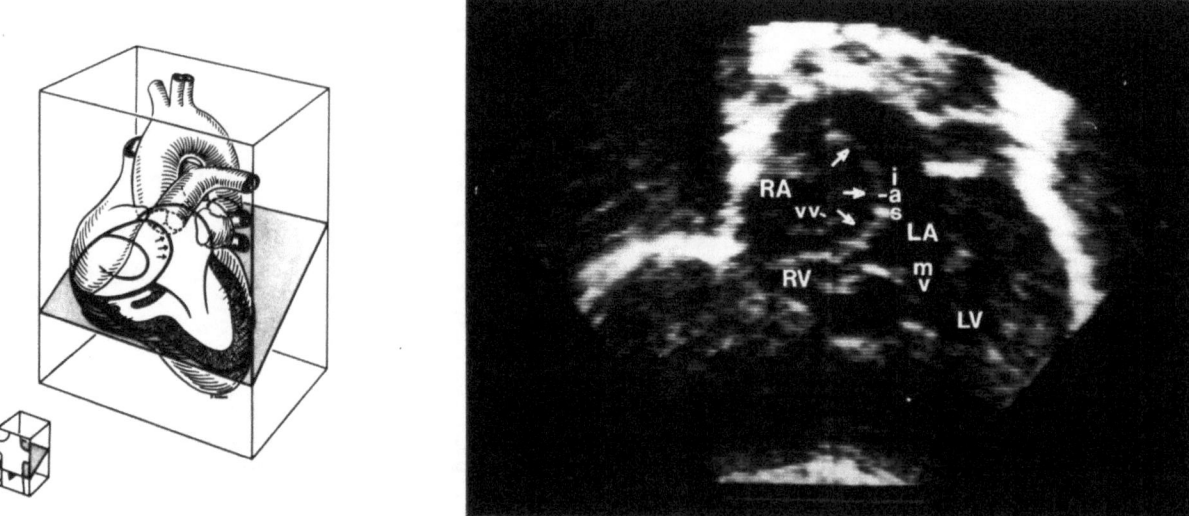

Figure 3.10. Subcostal four chamber two-dimensional echocardiogram of a patient with tricuspid atresia. The interatrial septum bulges as a whole to the left (arrows).
RA = right atrium, RV = right ventricle, vv = venous valve, ias = interatrial septum, LA = left atrium, mv = mitral valve, LV = left ventricle.

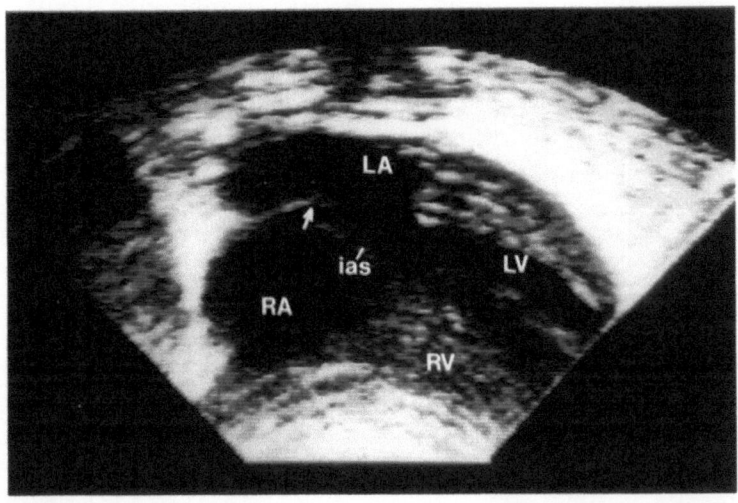

Figure 3.11. Subcostal four chamber two-dimensional echocardiogram of a patient with persistent foetal circulation. The region of the fossa ovalis bulges to the left (arrow).

    RA = right atrium, ias = interatrial septum, LA = left atrium, RV = right ventricle, LV = left ventricle.

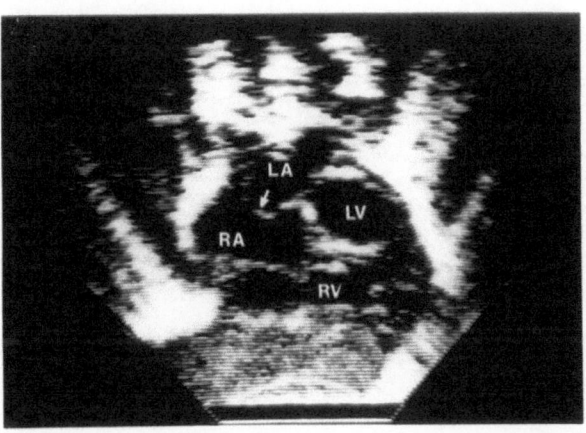

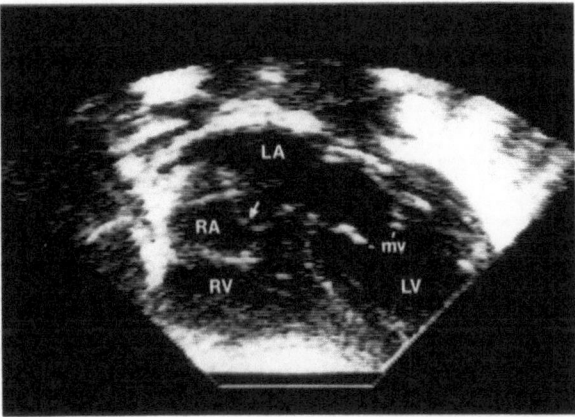

Figure 3.12. Subcostal four chamber two-dimensional echocardiogram of a patient with hypoplastic left heart syndrome. The interatrial septum is bulging to the right (arrow).

    RA = right atrium, LA = left atrium, RV = right ventricle, LV = left ventricle.

Figure 3.13. Subcostal four chamber two-dimensional echocardiogram of a patient with transposition of the great arteries and large ventricular septal defect. The interatrial septum is bulging to the right (arrow).

    RA = right atrium, RV = right ventricle, LA = left atrium, LV = left ventricle, mv = mitral valve.

4. ATRIOVENTRICULAR SEPTAL DEFECTS

The term atrioventricular septal defect is synonymous with endocardial cushion defect and persistent atrioventricular canal malformation. The essential feature of these defects is that the upper part of the inlet septum i.e. the atrioventricular septum has failed to develop (1). Consequently, the connection between the interventricular inlet septum and the ventral part of the interatrial septum is absent. Atrioventricular septal defects can roughly be divided into two main forms i.e. the partial and the complete defects.

Partial atrioventricular septal defects

Partial atrioventricular septal defects have two separate atrioventricular orifices whereby the tricuspid and mitral valves are attached at the same level to the crest of the deficient or scooped out interventricular septum. Because of this and the fact that the interatrial septum is not connected with the interventricular septum there is a ventrally located interatrial connection without an interventricular communication. This anomaly is also known as ostium primum defect or atrial septal defect of the primum type.

The clinical presentation of patients with partial atrioventricular septal defect is similar to that of patients with atrial septal defect with or without mitral incompetence. The mitral valve is always abnormal because it is composed of three components whereby the anterior leaflet consists of two parts. This may cause mitral incompetence. Hence, the combination of the auscultatory findings compatible with atrial septal defect and a high frequency pan-systolic murmur at the apex of the heart, caused by the mitral incompetence, is very suggestive of a partial atrioventricular septal defect. Left axis deviation on the electrocardiogram is seldom missing. The vectorcardiogram shows the superior orientation of the QRS loop and a counterclockwise inscription of the loop in the frontal plane.

Until recently cardiac catheterization and left ventricular angiocardiography were indispensable for confirmation of the diagnosis. In atrioventricular septal defects the frontal left ventricular angiogram shows the typical 'goose neck' deformity of the left ventricular outflow tract which is primarily caused by the abnormal attachments of the mitral valve. M-mode echocardiography has been of value for the diagnosis of partial atrioventricular septal defect and also for the differentiation of the complete forms. However, two-dimensional echocardiography provides the most accurate and detailed definition of the atrioventricular septal defects (2, 3).

Partial defects can easily be differentiated from a secundum atrial septal defect with mitral prolapse and from the different forms of the complete atrioventricular septal defect. The subcostal four chamber view (Figure 4.1) shows two important aspects of the partial atrioventricular septal defect i.e. the ventral atrial septal defect (ostium primum defect) and the attachment of the tricuspid and mitral valves at the same level to the crest of the scooped out ventricular inlet septum. The same features can also be visualized in the apical four chamber view (Figure 4.2). The subcostal longitudinal view of Figure 4.3 shows the left ventricular outflow tract in a partial atrioventricular septal defect. This echo view approximates the information gained from the frontal left ventricular angiogram. A continuity is present between the interventricular septum and the aorta. The lower wall of the left ventricular outflow tract is convex upwards and to the left causing an angle between the axis of the left ventricular outflow tract and that of the body of the left ventricle. This is an aspect of the typical goose neck appearance.

Another feature of the partial atrioventricular septal defect is the bipartition of the anterior mitral leaflet. In normal subjects the single anterior mitral leaflet moves in a direct antero-posterior direction. In the presence of a bipartition the right part of the leaflet opens to the right and the left part to the left. Therefore, the echo's of the anterior leaflets disappear out of view when visualized in a sagittal cross-section e.g. the long axis view. For the same reason the short axis view, at the level of the mitral valve, should be used to visualize the two parts of the anterior leaflet (4). In this view the mitral leaflets remain visible throughout the whole cardiac cycle (Figure 4.4 and 4.5).

Congenital mitral incompetence, through a bipartition in the anterior mitral leaflet, may rarely occur as an isolated lesion. The diagnosis can be confirmed by two-dimensional echocardiography alone (5).

Analysis of the mitral incompetence in partial atrioventricular septal defects is possible by left ventricular echocontrast injections during cardiac catheterization. Frequently the regurgitation is entirely directed from the left ventricle to the right atrium (Figure 4.6).

Complete atrioventricular septal defects

The essential feature of the complete atrioventricular septal defects is the presence of a common atrioventricular orifice between the atria and the ventricles in the absence of a connection between interatrial septum and the posterior interventricular inlet septum. The atrioventricular valve in this orifice consists of five leaflets. Two of them, the anterior and posterior bridging leaflets, are common to the right and left heart. They span the combined atrioventricular septal defect and are inserted into both ventricles. The interventricular part of the defect underneath the bridging leaflets is large causing equal pressures in the two ventricles.

Clinically, the complete atrioventricular defect behaves like a large ventricular septal defect with pulmonary hypertension. The patients are often dystrophic and in cardiac failure. Progressive pul-

monary vascular disease with increased pulmonary vascular resistance can be an early sequel of complete atrioventricular septal defects. To prevent this, early diagnosis is necessary to allow a corrective procedure in the first year of life. There is a striking association between the atrioventricular septal defect and Down's syndrome, particularly with the complete forms. In the complete forms the electrocardiogram shows left axis deviation and is compatible with biventricular hypertrophy.

Recognition of the two main types of complete atrioventricular septal defects is based on whether or not the chordae of the anterior bridging leaflet are tethered to the crest of the anterior part of the interventricular septum. If not, the defect is said to have a free floating anterior leaflet and belongs to the previously described Rastelli type C complete atrioventricular defect. If there is chordal insertion of the anterior bridging leaflet into the crest of the interventricular septum the defect is referred to as Rastelli type A (6). The posterior bridging leaflet is always connected by the chordae to the posterior part of the interventricular septum. Both types are exhibited diagrammatically in Figure 4.7. The atrioventricular valves are shown in an open position. If one considers the valves in a closed position it will be appreciated that the posterior bridging leaflet with its chordal insertions into the posterior septum can readily be visualized in the subcostal or the apical four chamber planes. The drawing of the Rastelli type A defect shows how the anterior bridging leaflet is connected by chordae to the anteriorly situated part of the scooped out interventricular septum. The presence or absence of the chordae will be obvious in the parasternal four chamber view which visualizes simultaneously the anterior bridging leaflet and the anterior part of the interventricular septum. This approach to the anterior and posterior leaflets is also adopted by Smallhorn and associates (3).

The subcostal and the parasternal four chamber views of a complete atrioventricular septal defect with a free floating anterior bridging leaflet (Rastelli type C) during systole are shown in Figure 4.8. The subcostal view clearly demonstrates that the posterior bridging leaflet is inserted by chordae into the right side of the crest of the interventricular septum and also into a robust papillary muscle which is situated next to the interventricular septum. The parasternal view shows the absence of connections between the anterior bridging leaflet and the crest of the anterior part of the interventricular septum. Therefore, the large interventricular communication beneath the anterior bridging leaflet can clearly be seen. The interventricular communication beneath the posterior bridging leaflet is located between the chordae. The diastolic frame of the subcostal four chamber view of Figure 4.8 is displayed in Figure 4.9. The atria and ventricles comprise one large cavity which allows mixing of the saturated and the desaturated blood.

The posterior bridging leaflet is sometimes tethered by many short chordae into the interventricular septum. This may obscure a potential interventricular communication (Figure 4.10). A left ventricular echocontrast injection may be necessary to determine the presence or absence of such a communication.

The subcostal and parasternal four chamber views of a complete atrioventricular septal defect in which both anterior and posterior bridging leaflets are inserted by chordae to the interventricular septum (Rastelli type A) are shown in Figure 4.11. The left ventricular echocontrast injection revealed hardly any communication beneath the posterior bridging leaflet. Figure 4.12 shows a marked L-R shunt beneath the anterior bridging leaflet.

The apical four chamber view of a complete atrioventricular septal defect after surgical repair is shown in Figure 4.13.

References

1. Van Mierop LHS: Pathology and pathogenesis of the common cardiac malformations. Cardiovascular clinics vol. 2.1. Brest AN, Downing D (eds.), Philadelphia, F.A. Davis Company, 27 – 60, 1970.
2. Hagler DJ, Tajik AJ, Seward JB, Mair DD, Ritter DG: Real-time wide-angle sector echocardiography: antrioventricular canal defects. Circulation 59:140 – 150, 1979.
3. Smallhorn JF, Tommasini G, Anderson RH, Macartney FJ: Assessment of atrioventricular septal defects by two-dimensional echocardiography. Br Heart J 47:109 – 121, 1982.
4. Beppu S et al. Mitral cleft in ostium primum atrial septal defect assessed by cross-sectional echocardiography. Circulation 62:1099 – 1107, 1980.
5. Smallhorn JF, de Leval M, Stark J, Somerville J, Taylor JFN, Anderson RH, Macartney FJ: Isolated anterior mitral cleft. Two-dimensional echocardiographic assessment and differentiation from 'clefts' associated with atrioventricular septal defect. Br Heart J 48:109 – 116, 1982.
6. Rastelli GC, Kirklin JW, Titus JL: Anatomical observations on complete form of persistent common atrioventricular canal with special reference to atrioventricular valves. Mayo Clin Proc 41:296 – 308, 1966.

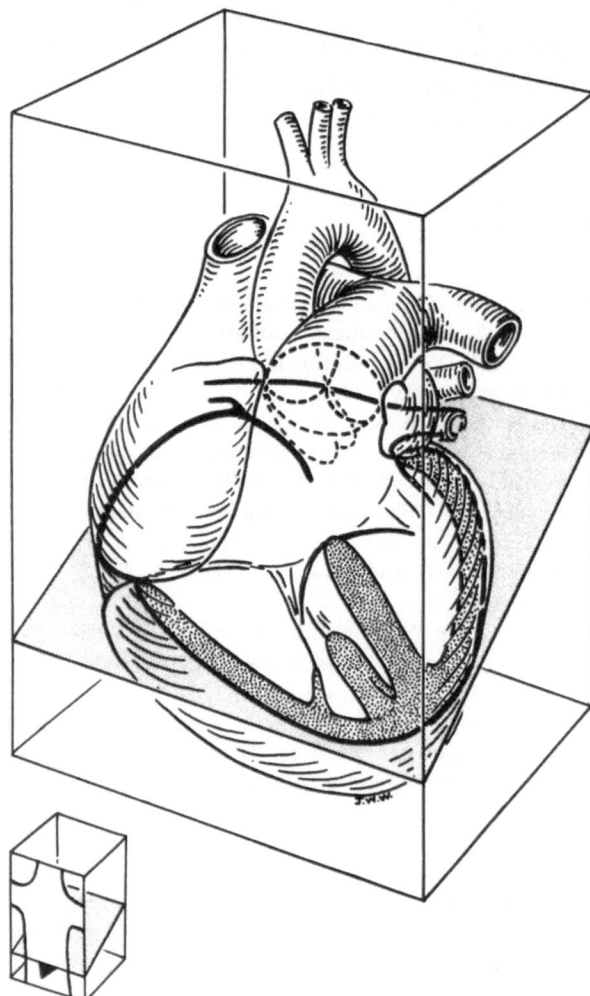

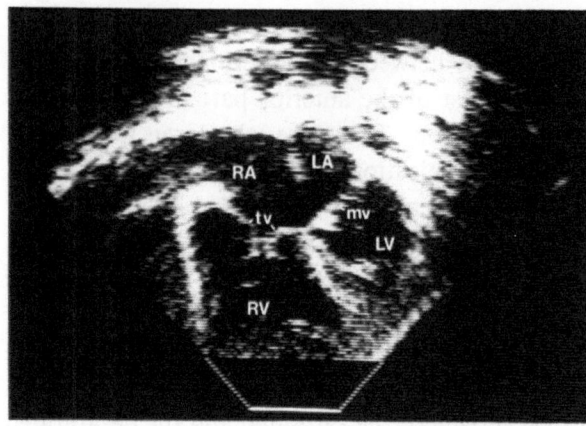

Figure 4.2. Apical four chamber two-dimensional echocardiogram of a patient with partial atrioventricular septal defect. In this case there is some malalignment between interatrial and interventricular septum. Two tricuspid valve leaflets are clearly visualized. The attachment of the septal leaflet of the tricuspid valve onto the crest of the interventricular septum is obvious.

RA = right atrium, LA = left atrium, tv = tricuspid valve, mv = mitral valve, RV = right ventricle, LV = left ventricle.

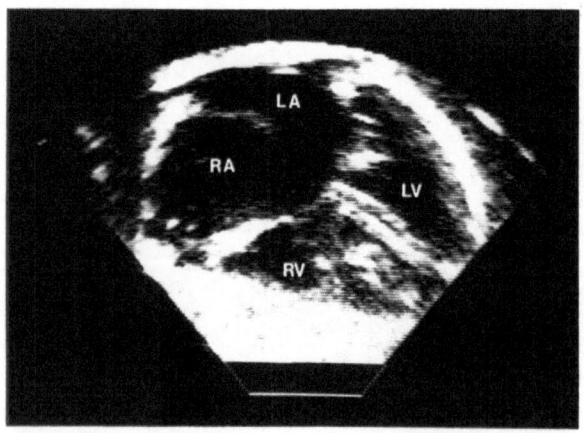

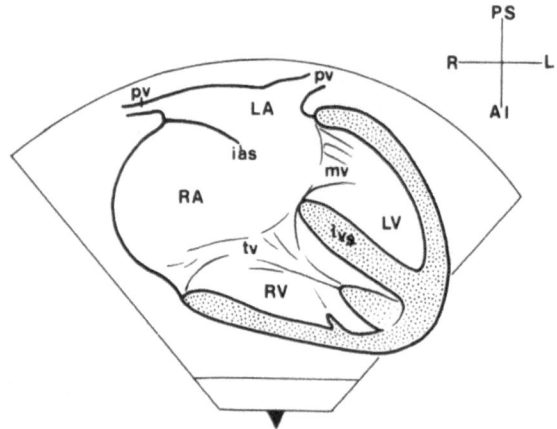

Figure 4.1. Subcostal four chamber two-dimensional echocardiogram of a patient with partial atrioventricular septal defect. There is a large ventral interatrial communication.

pv = pulmonary vein, LA = left atrium, RA = right atrium, ias = interatrial septum, mv = mitral valve, tv = tricuspid valve, ivs = interventricular septum, RV = right ventricle, LV = left ventricle.

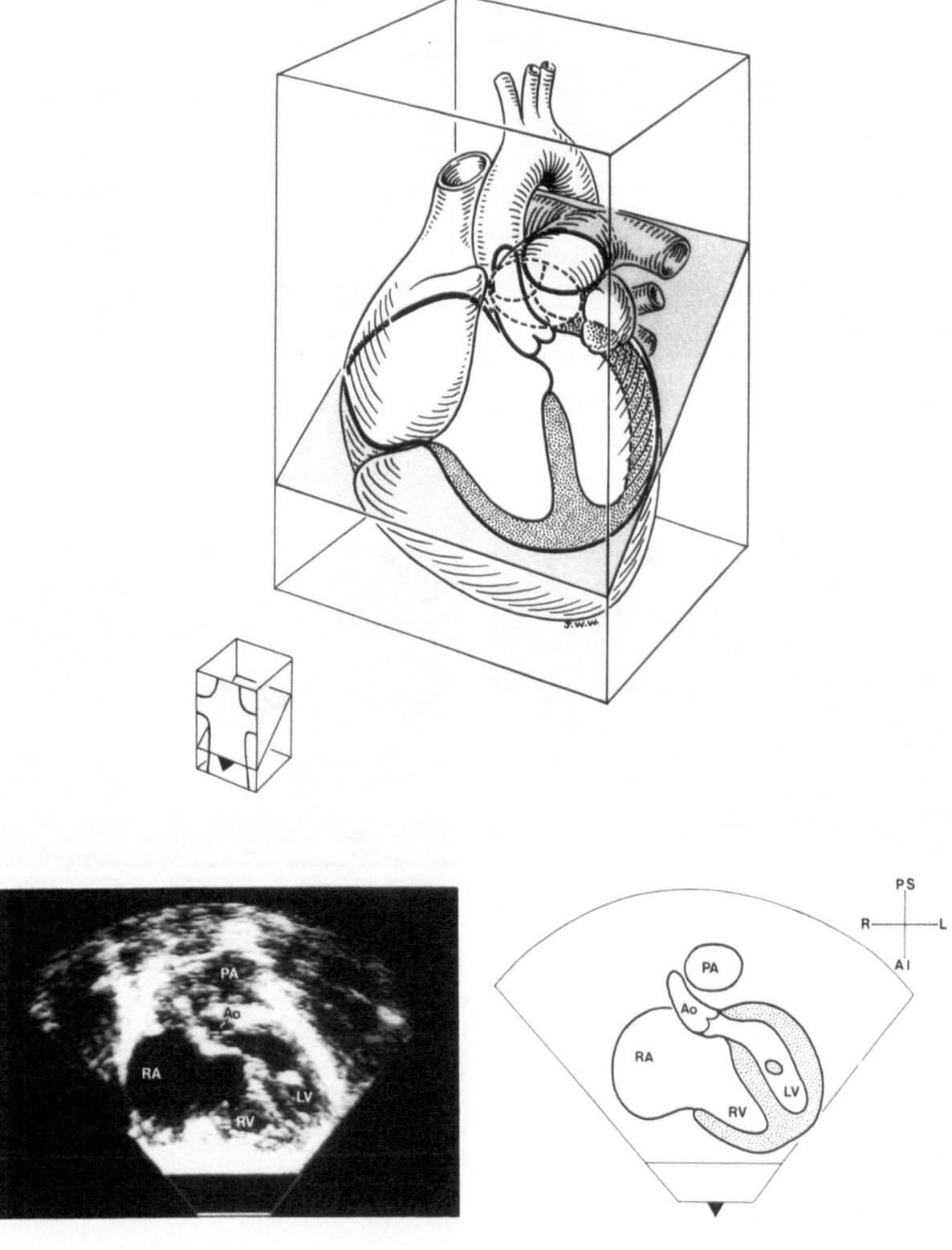

Figure 4.3. Subcostal longitudinal two-dimensional echocardiogram of the same patient as in Figure 4.1. In this diastolic still frame the opened tricuspid valve is not visible.

PA = pulmonary artery, Ao = aorta, RA = right atrium, RV = right ventricle, LV = left ventricle.

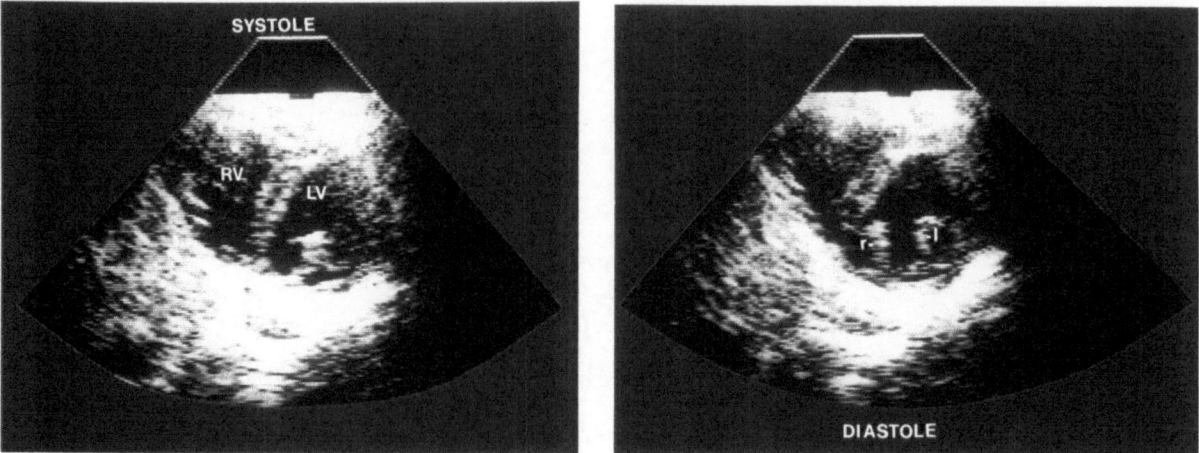

Figure 4.4. Parasternal short axis two-dimensional echocardiograms of a patient with partial atrioventricular septal defect showing the bipartition of the anterior mitral valve leaflet. In the systolic still frame the two parts are apposing each other and in diastole they are clearly separated.

RV = right ventricle, LV = left ventricle, r = right part of the anterior mitral valve leaflet, l = left part of the anterior mitral valve leaflet.

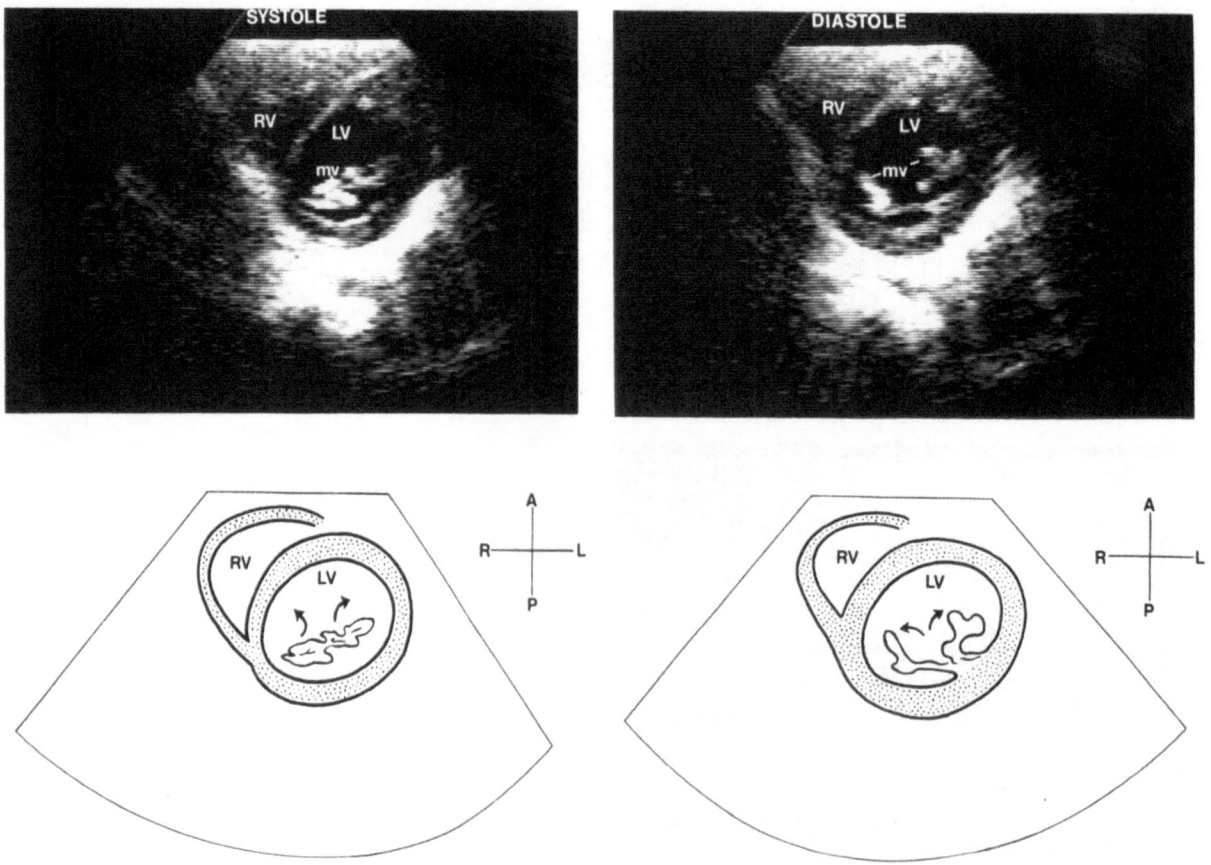

Figure 4.5. Parasternal short axis two-dimensional echocardiograms of a patient with partial atrioventricular septal defect who underwent a surgical correction. The two parts of the anterior mitral valve leaflet are partially joined by sutures near their attachment to the valve ring. The mitral valve appears deformed. The bipartition of the anterior leaflet remains clear during diastole.

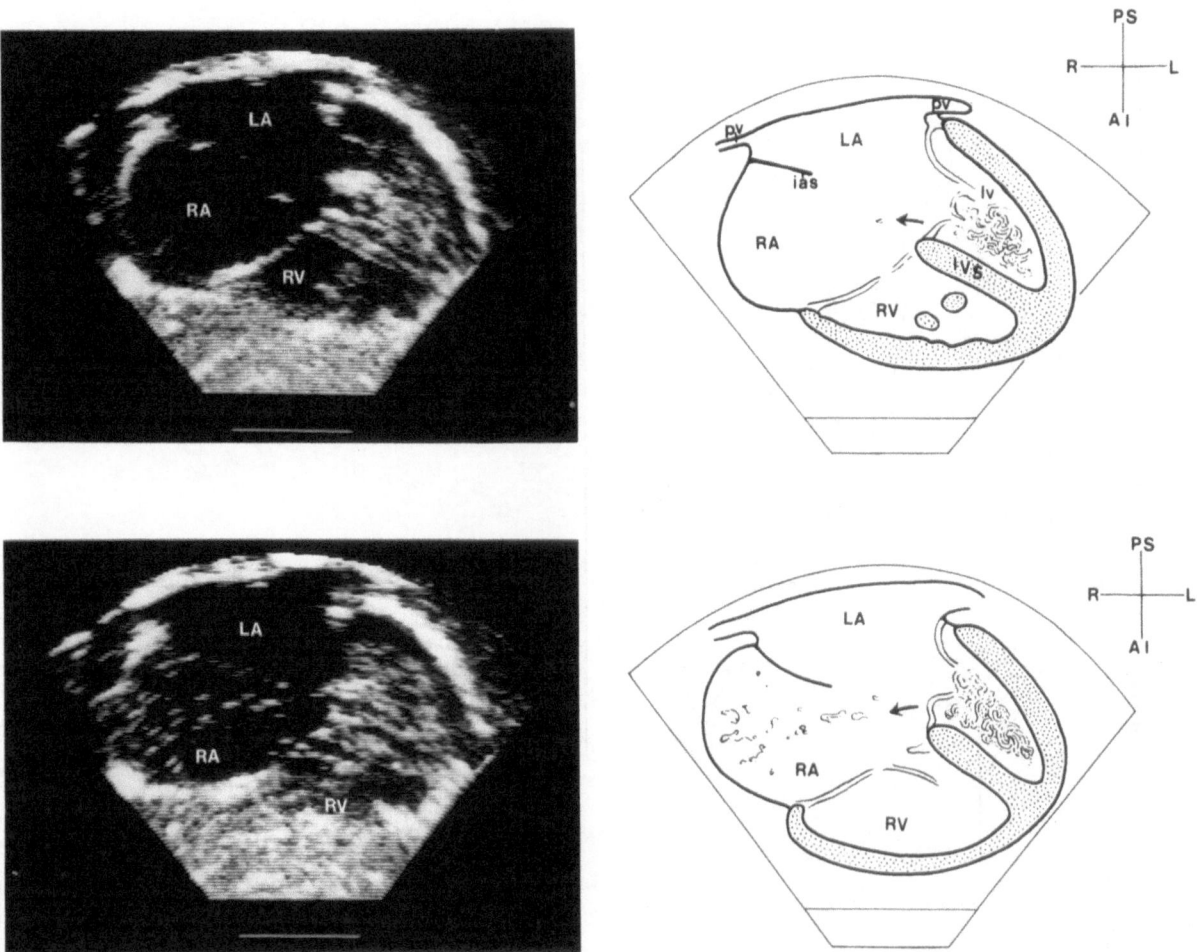

Figure 4.6. Subcostal four chamber two-dimensional echocardiograms of a patient with partial atrioventricular septal defect and mitral insufficiency. After the left ventricular echocontrast injection the left ventricle is filled (above). The regurgitant jet is directed towards the right atrium and contrast particles reach the right and posterior wall of the right atrium (below).

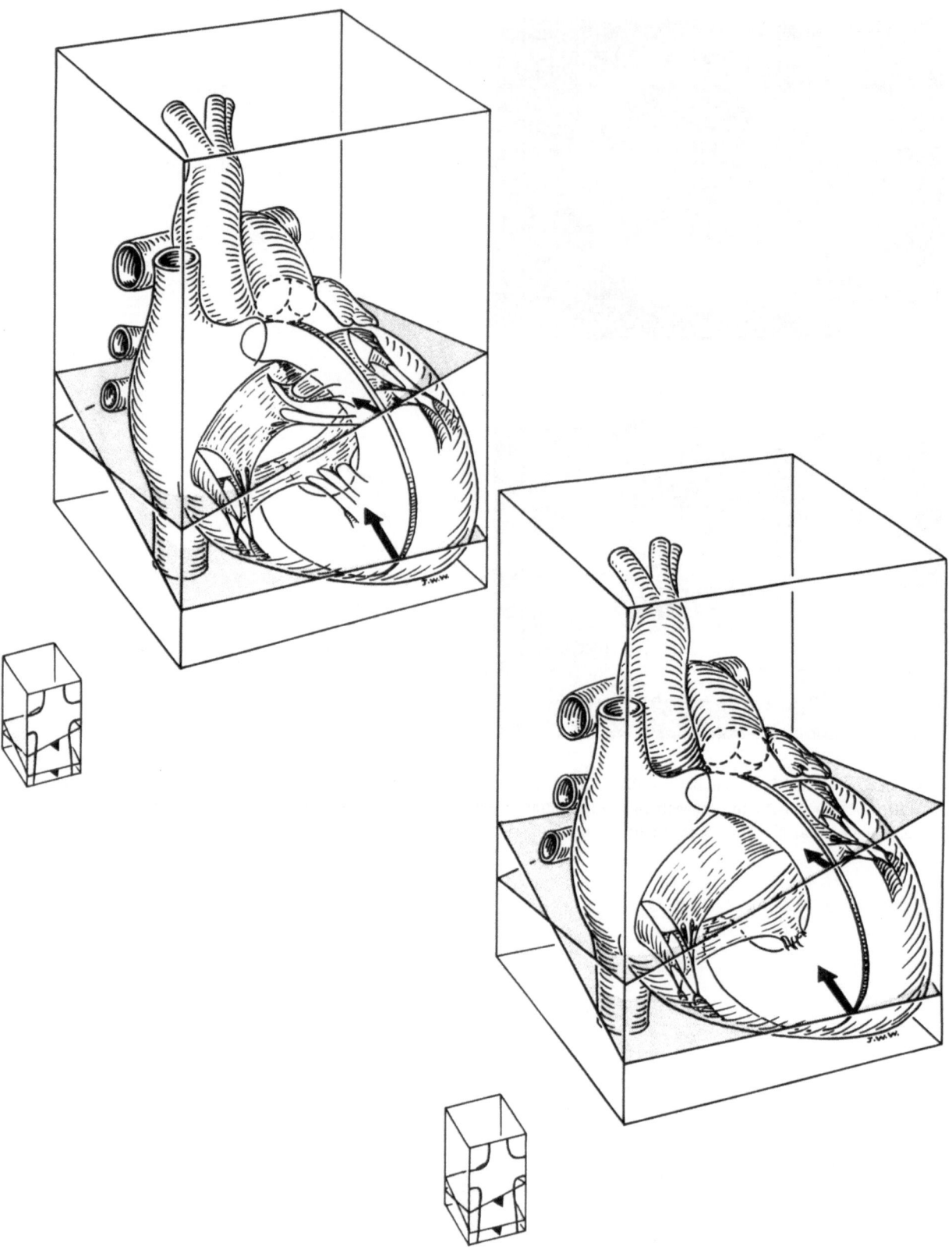

Figure 4.7. Drawings of complete atrioventricular septal defects. On the left the Rastelli type A in which the anterior bridging leaflet is connected with chordae to the anterior part of the interventricular septum. On the right the Rastelli type C with free floating anterior bridging leaflet. The plane with the larger black arrow represents the subcostal and the other plane the parasternal four chamber cross-sections.

61

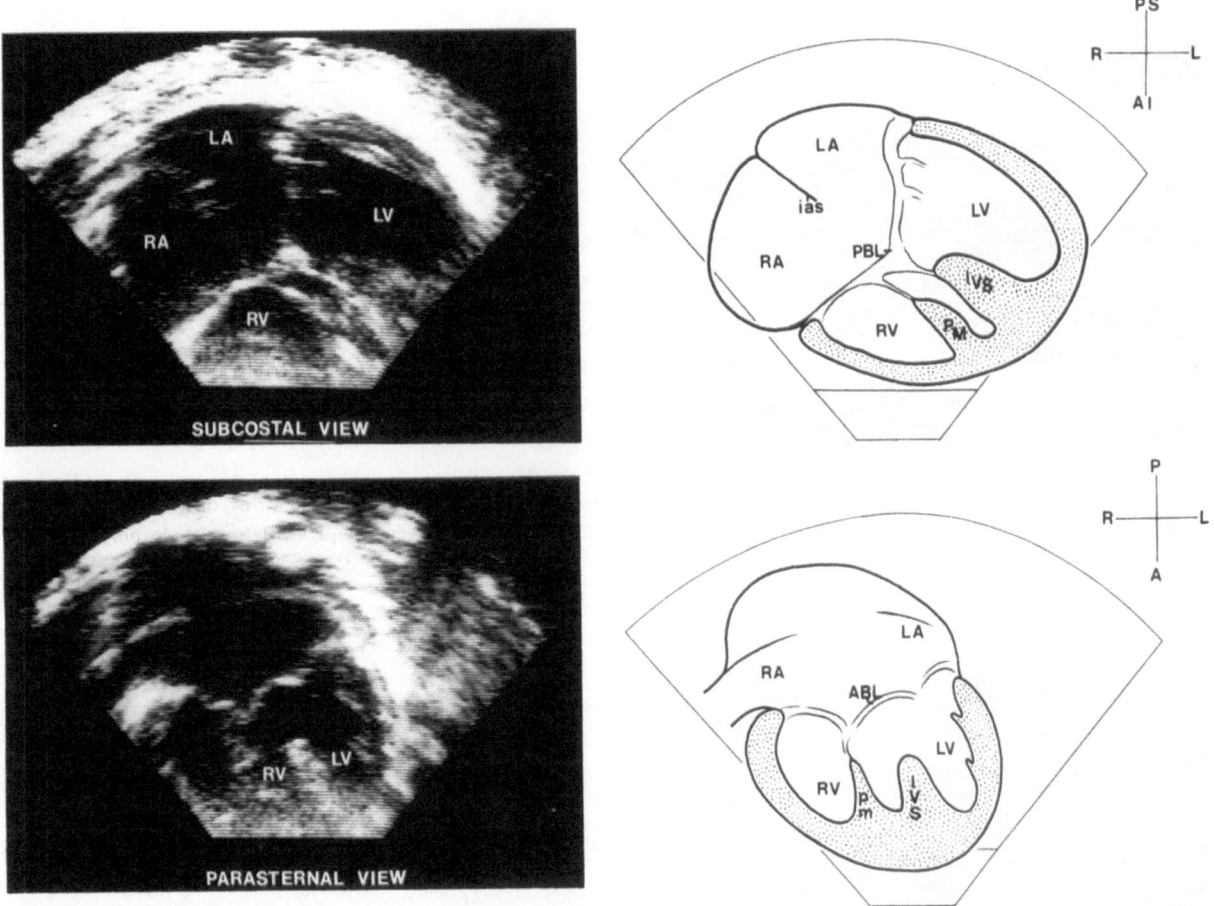

Figure 4.8. Four chamber two-dimensional echocardiograms of a patient with Rastelli type C complete atrioventricular septal defect.

LA = left atrium, RA = right atrium, ias = interatrial septum, PBL = posterior bridging leaflet, ABL = anterior bridging leaflet, RV = right ventricle, LV = left ventricle, PM, pm = papillary muscle, IVS = interventricular septum.

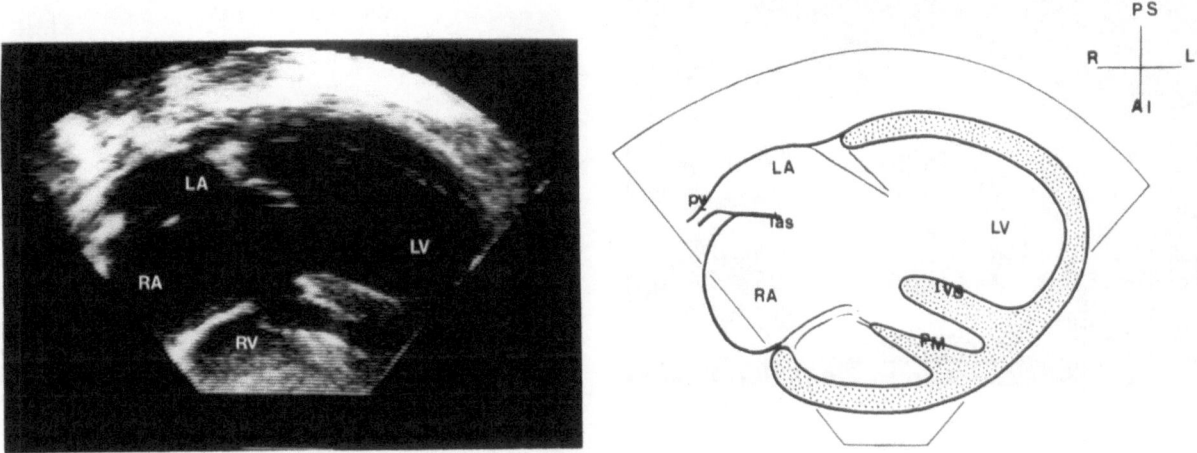

Figure 4.9. Subcostal four chamber view in diastole of the same patient as in Figure 4.8.

pv = pulmonary vein, ias = interatrial septum, LA = left atrium, RA = right atrium, LV = left ventricle, RV = right ventricle, *pm = papillary muscle*, IVS = interventricular septum.

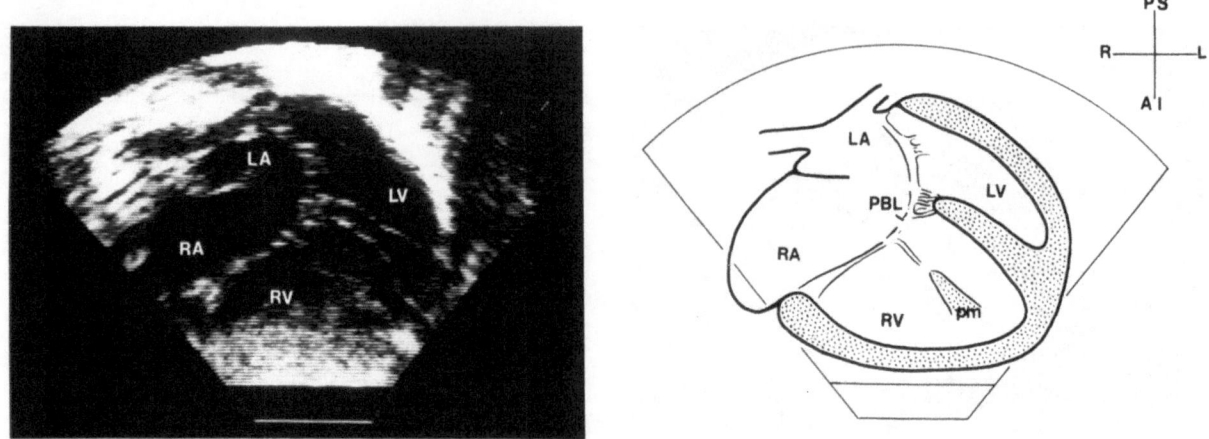

Figure 4.10. Subcostal four chamber two-dimensional echocardiogram of a patient with complete atrioventricular septal defect.
   RA = right atrium, LA = left atrium, PBL = posterior bridging leaflet, RV = right ventricle, LV = left ventricle, pm = papillary muscle.

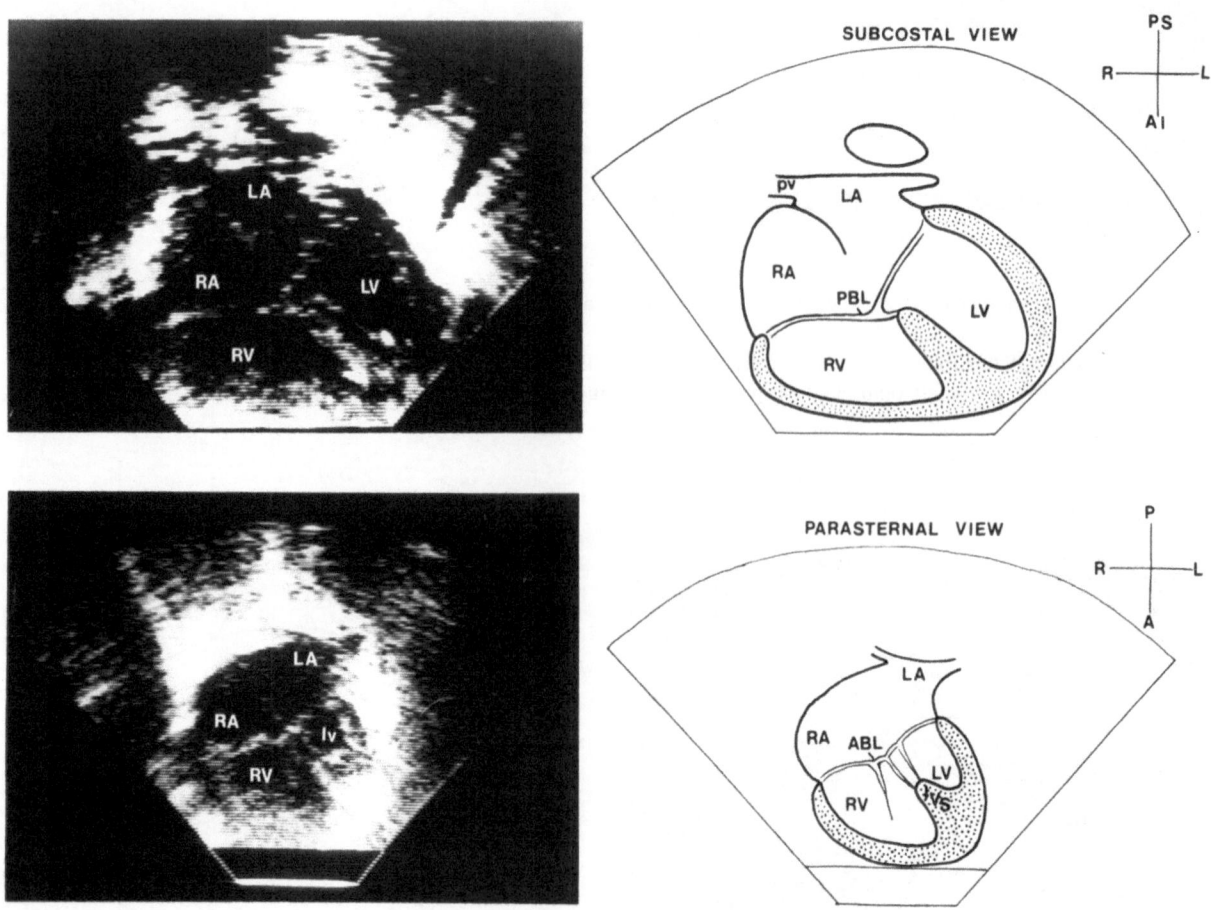

Figure 4.11. Four chamber two-dimensional echocardiograms of a patient with Rastelli type A complete atrioventricular septal defect.
   RA = right atrium, LA = left atrium, RV = right ventricle, LV, lv = left ventricle, pv = pulmonary vein, PBL = posterior bridging leaflet, ABL = anterior bridging leaflet, IVS = interventricular septum.

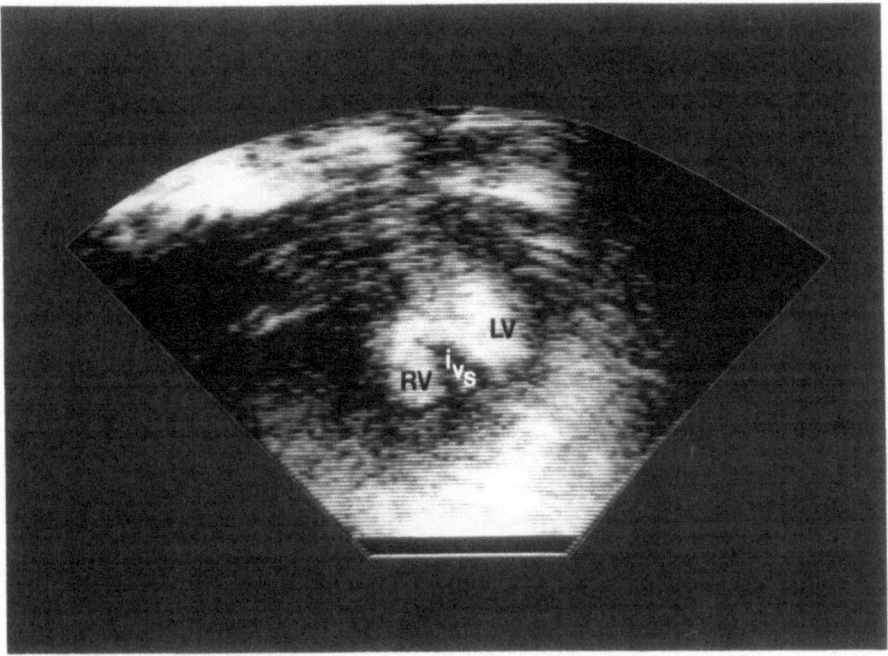

Figure 4.12. Parasternal four chamber view of the same patient as in Figure 4.11. After a left ventricular echocontrast injection the contrast passed from the left ventricle over the crest of the interventricular septum into the right ventricle.

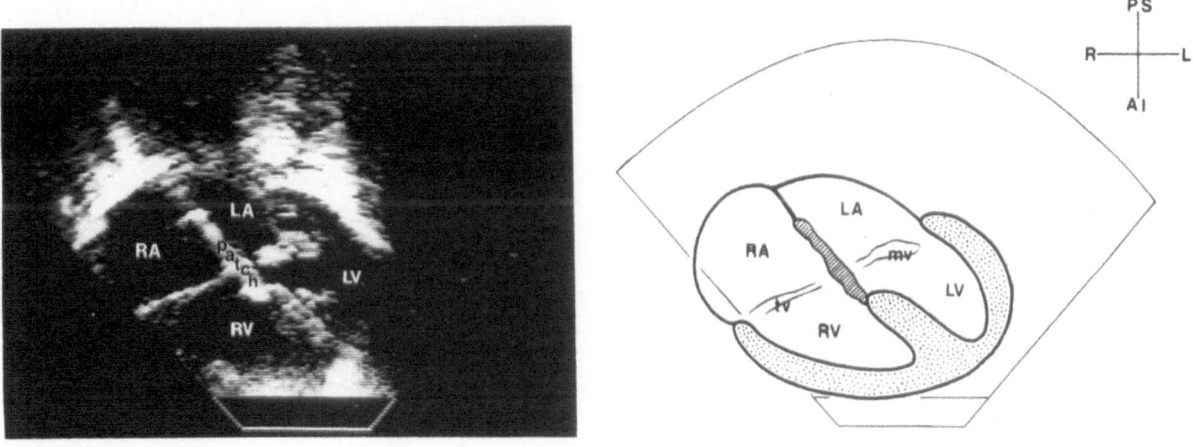

Figure 4.13. Apical four chamber two-dimensional echocardiogram of a patient with complete atrioventricular septal defect after surgical correction.

RA = right atrium, LA = left atrium, tv = tricuspid valve, mv = mitral valve, RV = right ventricle, LV = left ventricle.

5. DUCTUS ARTERIOSUS AND AORTO-PULMONARY WINDOW

The ductus arteriosus is a large channel through which blood flows from the main pulmonary artery to the descending aorta before birth. After birth the wall of the ductus contracts and closure usually occurs in the first few days of life.

Ductus arteriosus

Closure of the ductus is frequently delayed in preterm infants, particularly in association with respiratory distress. In these neonates there may be a predominant R-L, bidirectional or predominant L-R ductal shunt depending on the pulmonary vascular resistance. The L-R shunt normally becomes manifest clinically through a continuous murmur. The diastolic component of the murmur, however, is often missing in preterm infants. In these cases there may be a high-pitched systolic murmur difficult to differentiate from a ventricular septal defect, albeit, that its localisation is normally situated more superiorly. There is no murmur in the so-called silent ductus despite a large L-R shunt. In such a case a bounding precordial cardiac impulse and bounding peripheral pulses may be the only signs on physical examination. Two-dimensional echocardiography is valuable to detect ductal patency and to establish or refute the presence of additional cardiovascular disease.

It is often possible to visualize the ductus directly, especially in preterm infants. In these infants the ductus is commonly not even partially closed and the diameter is frequently as wide as the descending aorta. To detect the ductus the descending aorta and the main pulmonary artery should be imaged simultaneously. This is possible in a short axis view at the level of the great arteries whereby the bifurcation of the main pulmonary artery is visualized together with the transversely

cut descending aorta (see chapter 1, Figure 1.16). Sahn and Allen described the direct visualization of the ductus in this plane (1).

The ductus can also be looked for in a parasternal or subcostal sagittal plane, which displays the main pulmonary artery simultaneously with a longitudinal section of the descending aorta (see chapter 1, Figure 1.17). A parasternal view of a preterm infant with delayed closure of the ductus is shown in Figure 5.1. The ductus is demonstrated as a direct continuity between the most posterior part of the main pulmonary artery and the upper part of the descending aorta. The left atrium and the left ventricle are also seen in this cross-section. Therefore, it is the appropriate view to demonstrate a potential ductal R-L shunt by means of a peripheral venous contrast injection. An example of such a R-L ductal shunt can be seen in Figure 5.2. As the echocontrast does not enter the left atrium and the left ventricle, a concomitant R-L intracardiac shunt is excluded. The contrast entering the descending aorta is evidently caused by a R-L ductal shunt alone.

When there is also a R-L atrial shunt frame by frame analysis may reveal that echocontrast from the pulmonary artery enters the descending aorta before the atrially shunted contrast has passed the left ventricle. R-L ductal shunts are often seen in preterm infants with respiratory distress, however, they also occur in full-term infants. The condition is often referred to as persistent foetal circulation syndrome or persistent pulmonary hypertension of the newborn and is commonly associated with perinatal asphyxia.

A large L-R ductal shunt in preterm infants inevitably involves a significant volume overload of the left side of the heart. The increased left atrial and left ventricular dimensions are readily recognized echocardiographically. Left atrial dilatation increases the left atrium/aorta ratio. Typical diastolic flow patterns (reversed flow) in the main pulmonary artery, compatible with a L-R ductal shunt, may be demonstrated in these infants by echocardiography in combination with pulsed Doppler (2). In our experience the diagnosis of delayed closure of the ductus with a large L-R shunt in a preterm infant can accurately be established non-invasively by the combination of physical and two-dimensional echocardiographic investigations.

Persistent ductus arteriosus in full-term infants is rarely symptomatic because narrowing, to a certain extent, has nearly always taken place. In these cases the ductus forms a narrow channel allowing only a small L-R shunt. In these cases a typical continuous murmur is always present. It is a crescendo murmur up to the second heart sound and decrescendo during diastole indicating that the pressure in the pulmonary artery is lower than that in the aorta throughout the whole cardiac cycle. Such a narrow ductus cannot be demonstrated directly by echocardiography. The abnormal diastolic flow pattern in the pulmonary artery can be registered by echo Doppler.

Occasionally the L-R ductal shunt is large and may cause symptoms of cardiac failure. In the presence of a wide interarterial channel the large L-R shunt may cause pulmonary hypertension. In these cases the diastolic component of the murmur may also be missing or shortened. Echocardiography reveals the volume overload of the left heart in the presence of an intact interventricular septum. Direct visualization of the ductus is often possible in these patients.

Figure 5.3 shows the two-dimensional echocardiograms of a 6 months old infant with a large L-R ductal shunt. The ductus is visualized in the parasternal sagittal view and in the short axis view at the level of the great arteries. Similar views with a catheter through the ductus are also exhibited in Figure 5.3 and 5.4. In the short axis view the ductus is seen as a third posterior branch of the main pulmonary artery, which is particularly clear in Figure 5.5.

Ductus arteriosus in transposition of the great arteries

Patency of a ductus can also be demonstrated by two-dimensional echocardiography in transposition of the great arteries. In the subcostal longitudinal view (Figure 5.6) the left ventricle gives rise to the main pulmonary artery which can be identified by its bifurcation. A tortuous ductus originates at the site of the origin of the left pulmonary artery and clearly communicates with the transversely cut descending aorta. In a subcostal sagittal view (Figure 5.7) another case is demonstrated. This patient also had a subpulmonary stenosis caused by accessory mitral valve tissue. A venous contrast injection opacified in sequence the right ventricle, descending aorta and retrograde through the ductus the pulmonary artery (figure 5.8). A R-L intracardiac shunt was excluded because the echocontrast did not enter the left atrium and the left ventricle.

Aorto-pulmonary window

Aorto-pulmonary window is also called aorto-pulmonary septal defect or partial truncus arteriosus. A defect of the aorto-pulmonary septum causes a communication between the ascending aorta and the main pulmonary artery. The incidence of aorto-pulmonary window is markedly lower than that of persistent ductus arteriosus. Most defects are large enough to equalize pressures in aorta and pulmonary artery. The anomaly has to be differentiated from large persistent ductus arteriosus because cardio-pulmonary bypass is necessary for surgical closure. In our patients with isolated aorto-pulmonary window the diagnosis could be established with two-dimensional echocardiography. Valuable information may be gained from the short axis views at great artery level (3). In our cases the normal circle-sausage appearance of the aorta and right ventricular outflow tract with pulmonary artery was absent. Indeed, at semilunar valve level there were two circles in a right posterior/left anterior or in a more side by side relation. By shifting the transducer more cranially the fenestration could be visualized (Figure 5.9). The subcostal views can also be used. Smallhorn et al. also found suprasternal cuts useful (4).

The subcostal view (Figure 5.10) exhibits the pulmonary artery slightly anterior to the aorta. Only a small part of the proximal aorto-pulmonary septum is intact. The large deficiency of the distal part is obvious.

References

1. Sahn DJ, Allen HD: Real-time cross-sectional echocardiographic imaging and measurement of the patent ductus arteriosus in infants and children. Circulation 58:343 – 354, 1978.
2. Stevenson JG, Kawabori I, Guntheroth WG: Non-invasive detection of pulmonary hypertension in patent ductus arteriosus by pulsed Doppler echocardiography. Circulation 60:355 – 359, 1979.
3. Satomi G, Nakamura K, Imay Y, Takao A: Two-dimensional echocardiographic diagnosis of aorticopulmonary window. Br Heart J 43:351 – 356, 1980.
4. Smallhorn JF, Anderson RH, Macartney FJ: Two-dimensional echocardiographic assessment of communications between ascending aorta and pulmonary trunk or individual pulmonary arteries. Br Heart J 47:563 – 572, 1982.

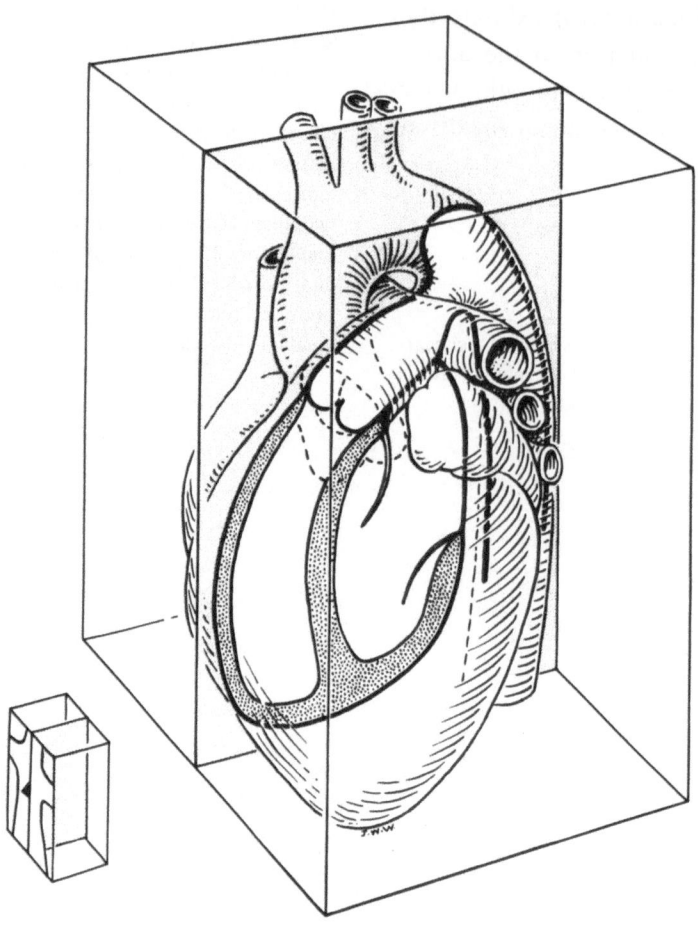

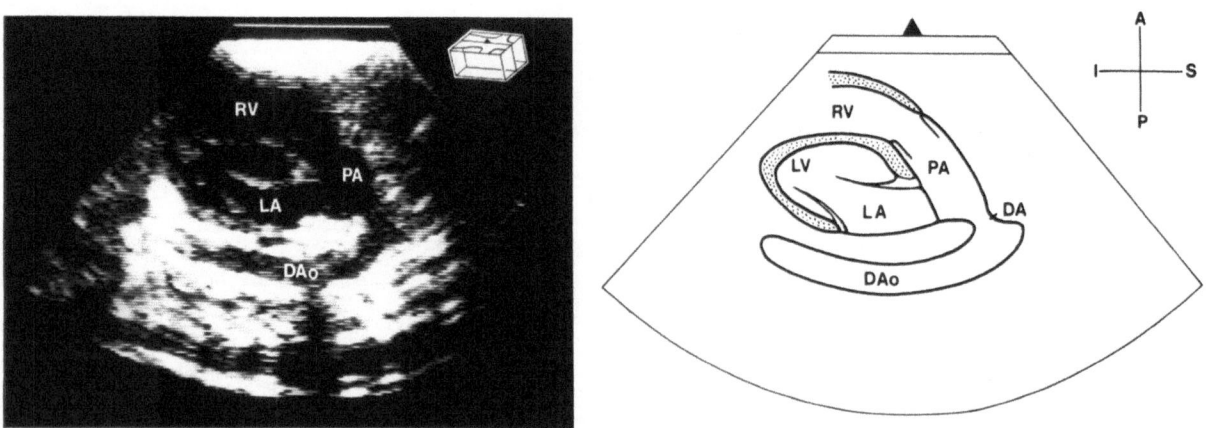

Figure 5.1. Parasternal sagittal two-dimensional echocardiogram of a preterm infant with delayed closure of the ductus arteriosus. The ductus is visualized in the plane of the pulmonary artery and descending aorta.

RV = right ventricle, PA = pulmonary artery, LV = left ventricle, LA = left atrium, DAo = descending aorta, DA = ductus arteriosus.

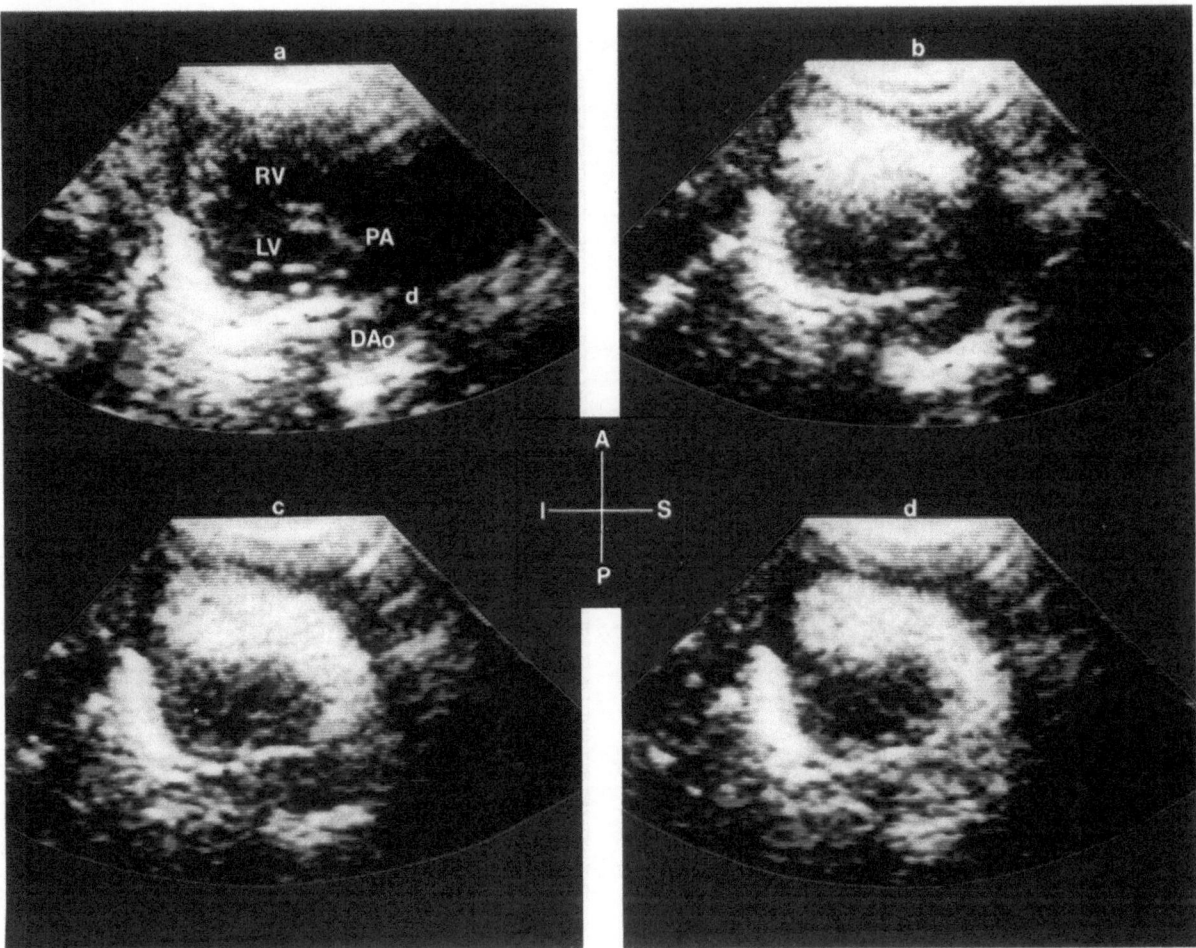

Figure 5.2. Parasternal sagittal two-dimensional echocardiograms before (a) and after (b, c, d) a venous echocontrast injection. The contrast firstly appears in the right ventricle (b) and passes into the pulmonary artery (c). In panel d the descending aorta is filled through the ductus arteriosus. The left ventricle is still free of contrast.

RV = right ventricle, LV = left ventricle, PA = pulmonary artery, d = ductus, DAo = descending aorta.

SAGITTAL VIEW

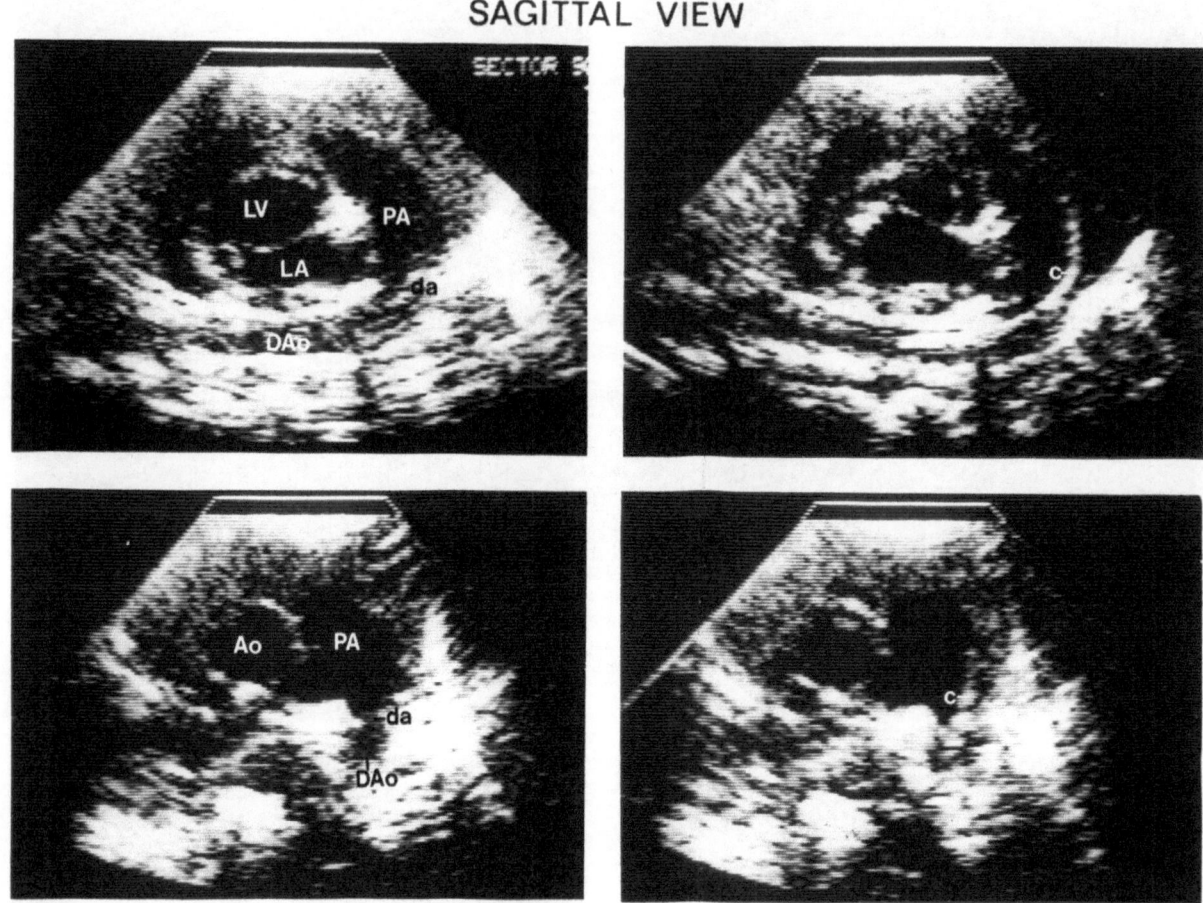

SHORT AXIS VIEW

Figure 5.3. Parasternal two-dimensional echocardiograms of a six months-old infant with persistent ductus arteriosus.
   LV = left ventricle, PA = pulmonary artery, LA = left atrium, DAo = descending aorta, da = ductus arteriosus, c = catheter.
For diagrams see Figure 5.4.

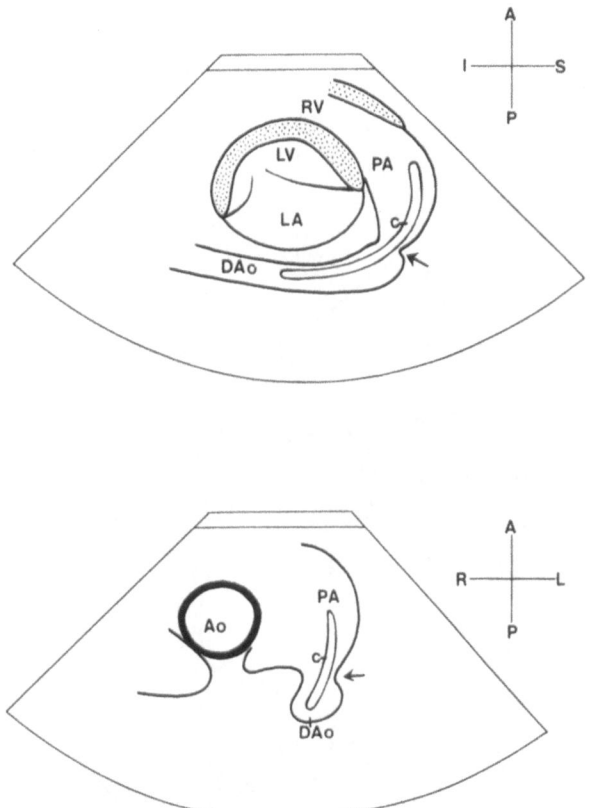

Figure 5.4. Diagrams belonging to Figure 5.3. Arrows indicate the site of the ductus.
RV = right ventricle, LV = left ventricle, PA = pulmonary artery, LA = left atrium, DAo = descending aorta, c = catheter.

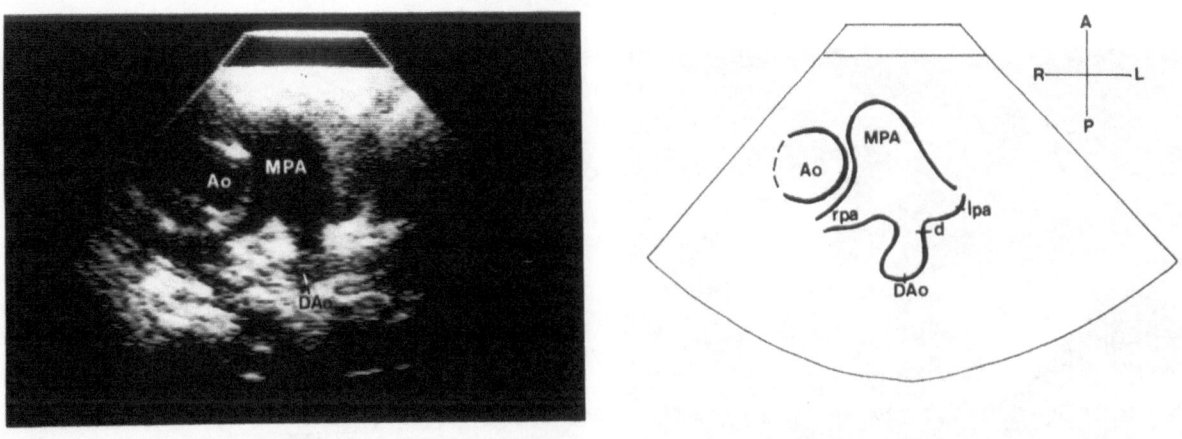

Figure 5.5. Parasternal short axis view showing 'the three branches' of the main pulmonary artery in a patient with persistent ductus arteriosus.
MPA = main pulmonary artery, Ao = aorta, DAo = descending aorta, d = ductus arteriosus, rpa = right pulmonary artery, lpa = left pulmonary artery.

72

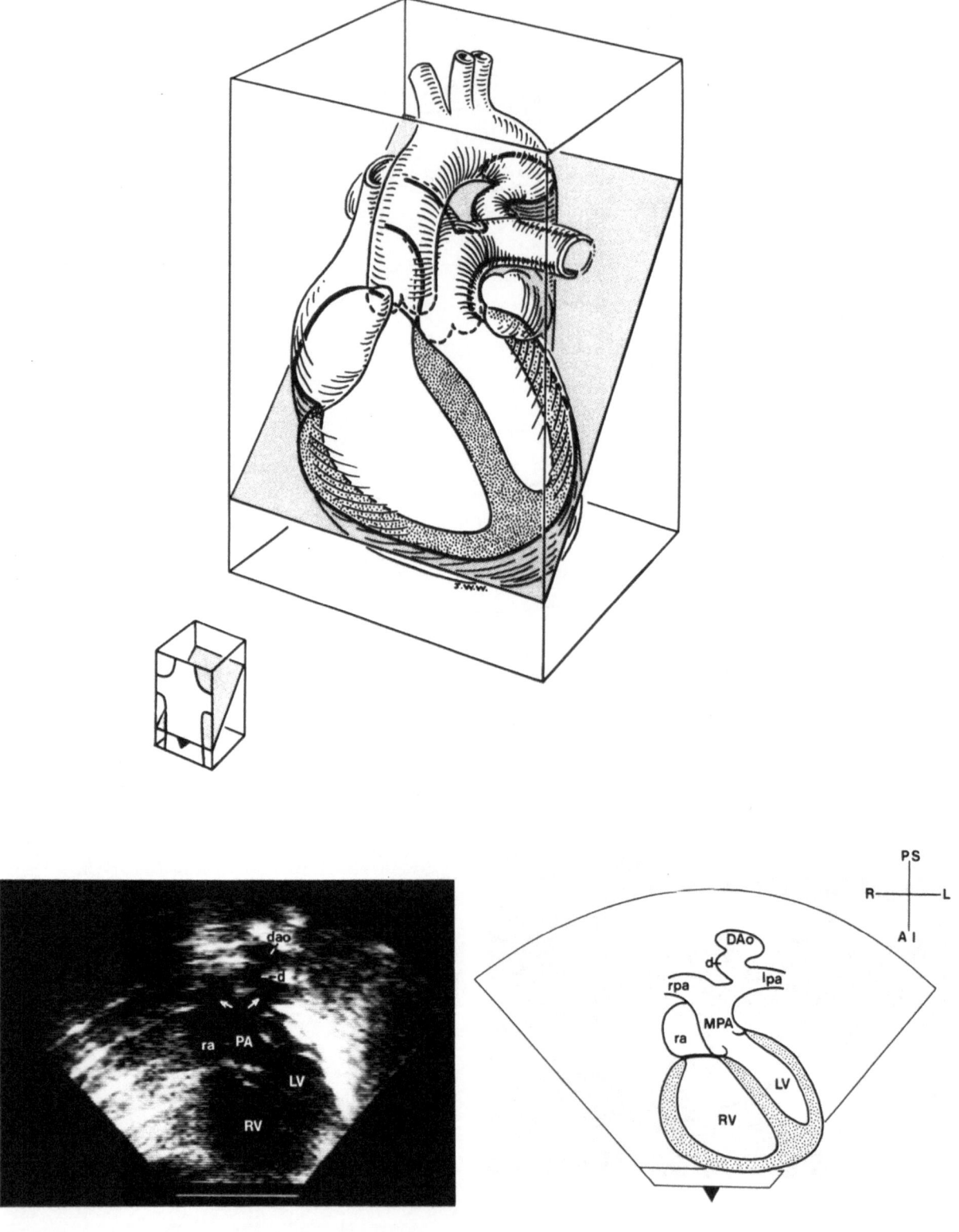

Figure 5.6. Subcostal longitudinal two-dimensional echocardiogram of a patient with transposition of the great arteries showing patency of the ductus arteriosus.

DAo, dao = descending aorta, d = ductus arteriosus, PA = pulmonary artery, MPA = main pulmonary artery, rpa = right pulmonary artery, lpa = left pulmonary artery, ra = right atrium, rv = right ventricle, RV = right ventricle, LV = left ventricle.

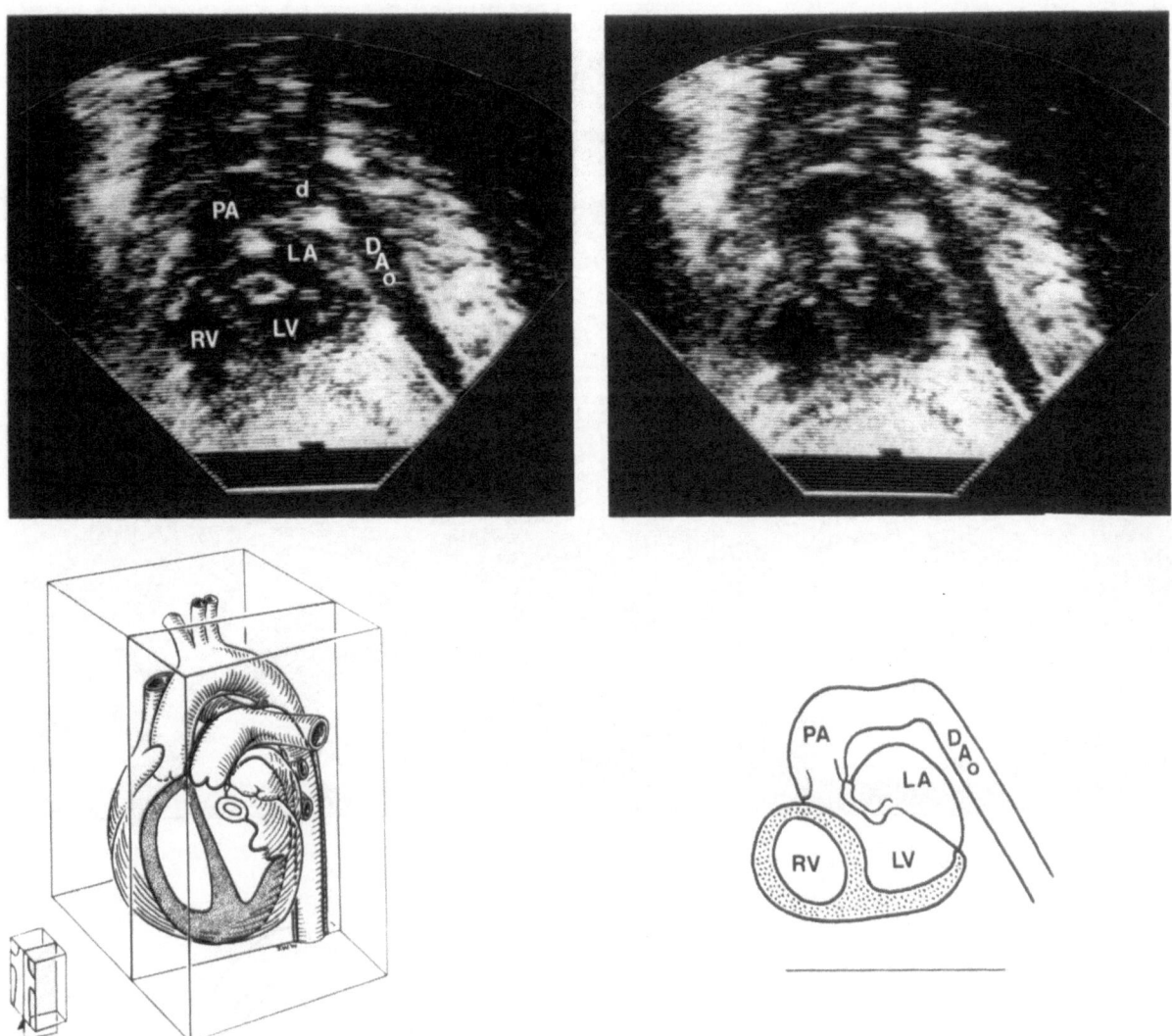

Figure 5.7. Subcostal sagittal two-dimensional echocardiograms of a patient with transposition of the great arteries, ductus arteriosus and a subpulmonic stenosis caused by accessory mitral valve tissue. The left still frame is taken in diastole and the right one in systole.

PA = pulmonary artery, RV = right ventricle, LV = left ventricle, LA = left atrium, DAo = descending aorta, d = ductus arteriosus.

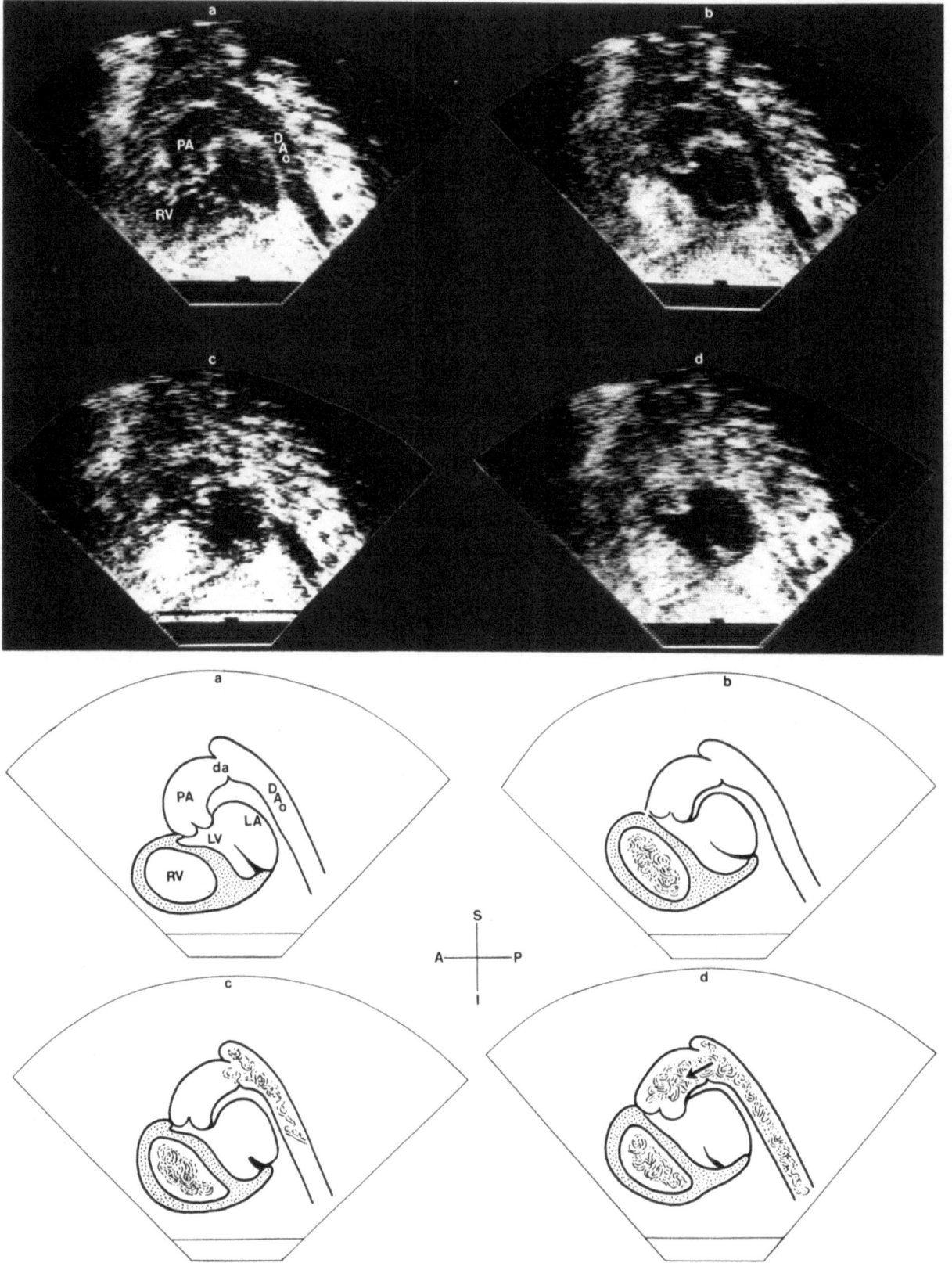

Figure 5.8. Subcostal sagittal two-dimensional echocardiograms of the same patient as in Figure 5.7. After a venous contrast injection the right ventricle is clearly opacified (b). In pannel c the contrast has appeared in the descending aorta and in d the main pulmonary artery is retrogradely filled through the ductus arteriosus.

RV = right ventricle, LV = left ventricle, LA = left atrium, PA = pulmonary artery, DAo = descending aorta, da = ductus arteriosus.

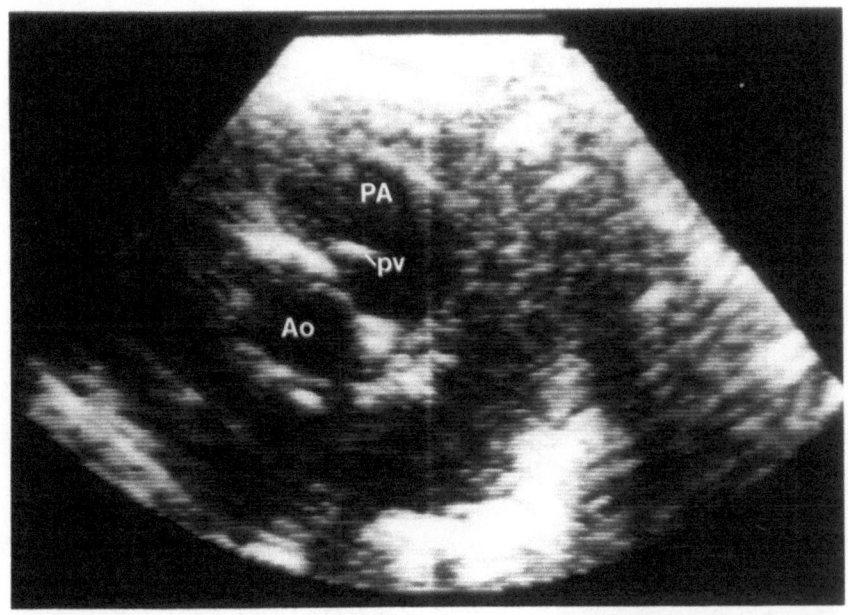

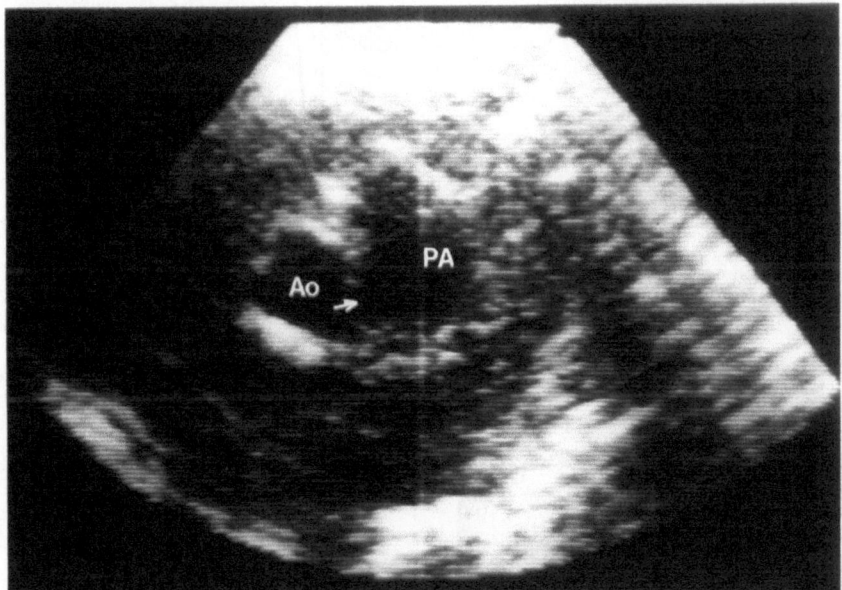

Figure 5.9. Parasternal short axis two-dimensional echocardiogram of a patient with a large aortopulmonary window. At pulmonary valve level (upper panel) the aorto-pulmonary septum is intact. Superior to the valve the communication between aorta and pulmonary artery is visualized (arrow, lower panel).

PA = pulmonary artery, Ao = aorta, pv = pulmonary valve.

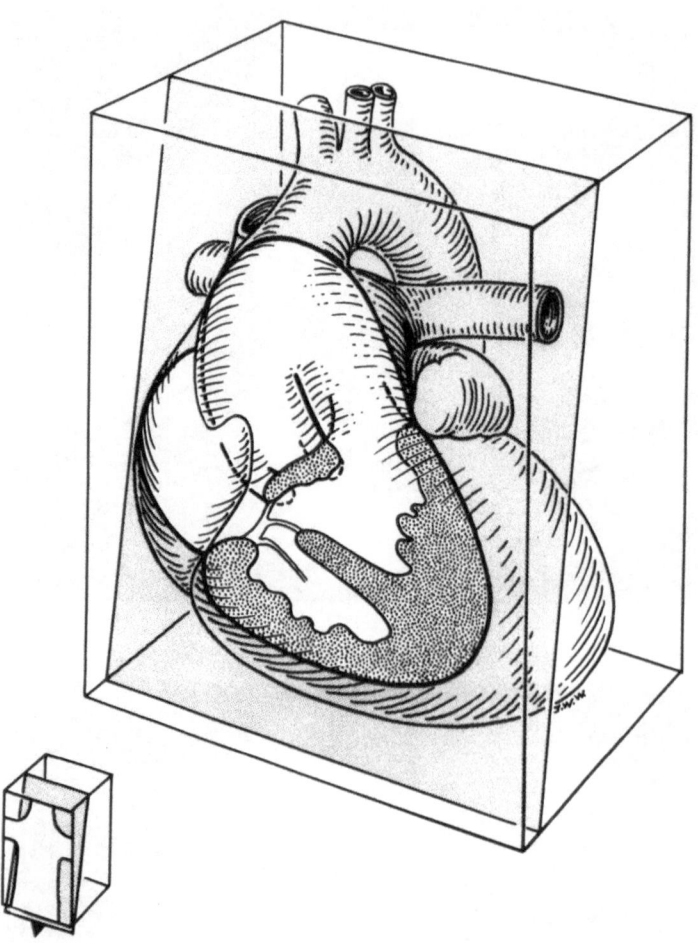

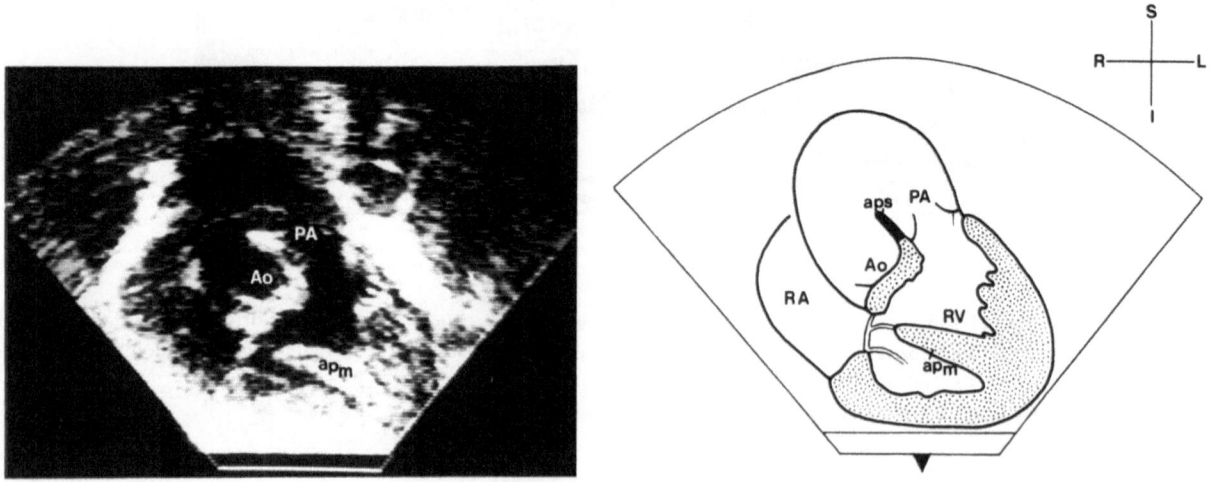

Figure 5.10. Subcostal frontal two-dimensional echocardiogram of a patient with a large aorto-pulmonary window.

Ao = aorta, PA = pulmonary artery, apm = anterior papillary muscle, aps = aorto-pulmonary septum, RA = right atrium, RV = right ventricle.

6. PULMONARY VALVE STENOSIS

Severe pulmonary valve stenosis causing symptoms of cardiac failure in the first months of life can be accurately diagnosed by non-invasive techniques. Auscultation reveals a harsh systolic ejection murmur at the left parasternal area. In the presence of cardiac failure this murmur may be absent and there may a high-pitched murmur caused by secondary tricuspid incompetence. The severe and fixed outflow obstruction of the right ventricle causes progressive right ventricular hypertrophy with markedly elevated diastolic pressures in the right side of the heart. Cyanosis may be present due to a concomitant R-L atrial shunt. The electrocardiogram is compatible with severe right ventricular hypertrophy. Chest X-ray may reveal normal or diminished pulmonary vascular markings.

The diagnosis can be confirmed by two-dimensional echocardiographic investigation. Other structural cardiac defects giving rise to cyanosis can be discarded. The two-dimensional echocardiogram will reveal the right ventricular hypertrophy and the abnormal pulmonary valve. Figure 6.1 and 6.2 show several views of a patient with severe pulmonary valve stenosis. The subcostal four chamber view reveals the bulging of the atrial septum to the left indicating that the pressure in the right atrium exceeds that of the left. The R-L atrial shunt can be verified by venous echocontrast injections. The globular shape and extremely thickened wall of the right ventricle are visualized in the long axis view. The left ventricle is flattened and its cavity obliterated during systole. This is indicative of suprasystemic right ventricular pressure. The short axis view, at the level of the great arteries, reveals a well developed pulmonary artery up to and just beyond the bifurcation. Ultrasound does not visualize the pulmonary artery much beyond the bifurcation, therefore a peripheral stenosis cannot be excluded. The closed pulmonary valve produces a dense echoshadow indicative of a thickened valve. Weyman and associates have described the visualisation of the dome-shaped valve on the two-dimensional echocardiogram during systole (1). In our experience it is more difficult to show the dome-shape of a stenotic pulmonary valve than that of a stenotic aortic valve. Nevertheless, this difficulty does not interfere with the accurate diagnosis of pulmonary valve stenosis and we have learned that cardiac catheterization is not needed to establish the anatomical features of this lesion.

Figure 6.3 shows the systolic doming of the pulmonary valve in a patient with pulmonary valve stenosis. The interventricular septum is convex to the right, therefore, the pressure in the right ventricle is lower than that in the left ventricle. The thickness of the walls of the right and left ventricle is almost equal. In mild to moderate pulmonary valve stenosis the two-dimensional echocardiogram may be of little or no diagnostic value because the abnormality of the pulmonary valve and the right ventricular hypertrophy may be difficult to recognize. The leftward convexity of the interatrial and interventricular septum described earlier is absent. In these cases physical examination and phonocardiography will yield the diagnostic information.

References

1. Weyman AE, Hurwitz RA, Girod DA, Dillon JC, Feigenbaum H, Green D: Cross-sectional echocardiographic visualisation of the stenotic pulmonary valve. Circulation 56:769–774, 1977.

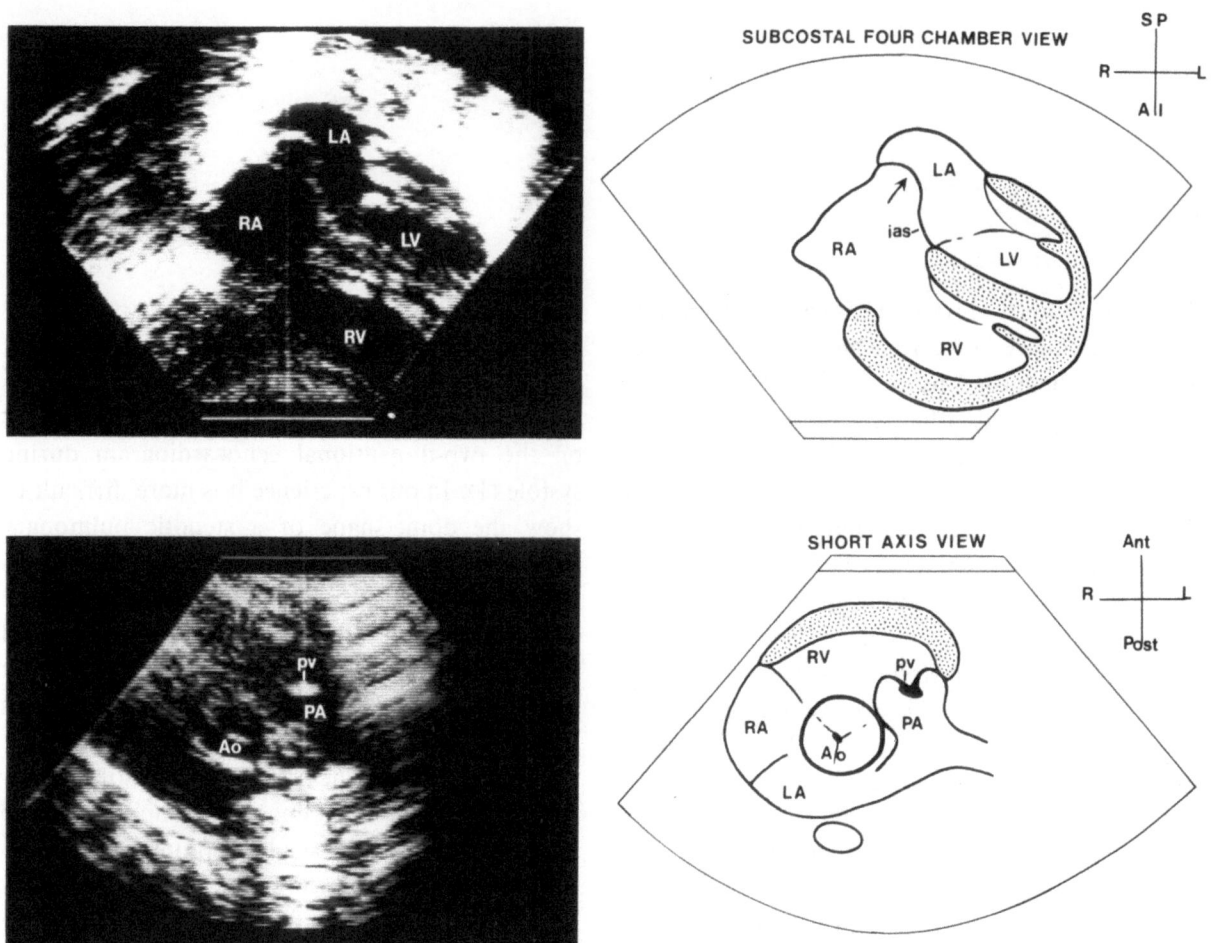

Figure 6.1. Two-dimensional echocardiograms of a patient with severe valvular pulmonary stenosis. The four chamber view discloses the bulging of the atrial septum to the left. The short axis view shows a thickened pulmonary valve echo in a normal sized valve ring.

RA = right atrium, ias = interatrial septum, LA = left atrium, LV = left ventricle, RV = right ventricle, Ao = aorta, PA = pulmonary artery, pv = pulmonary valve.

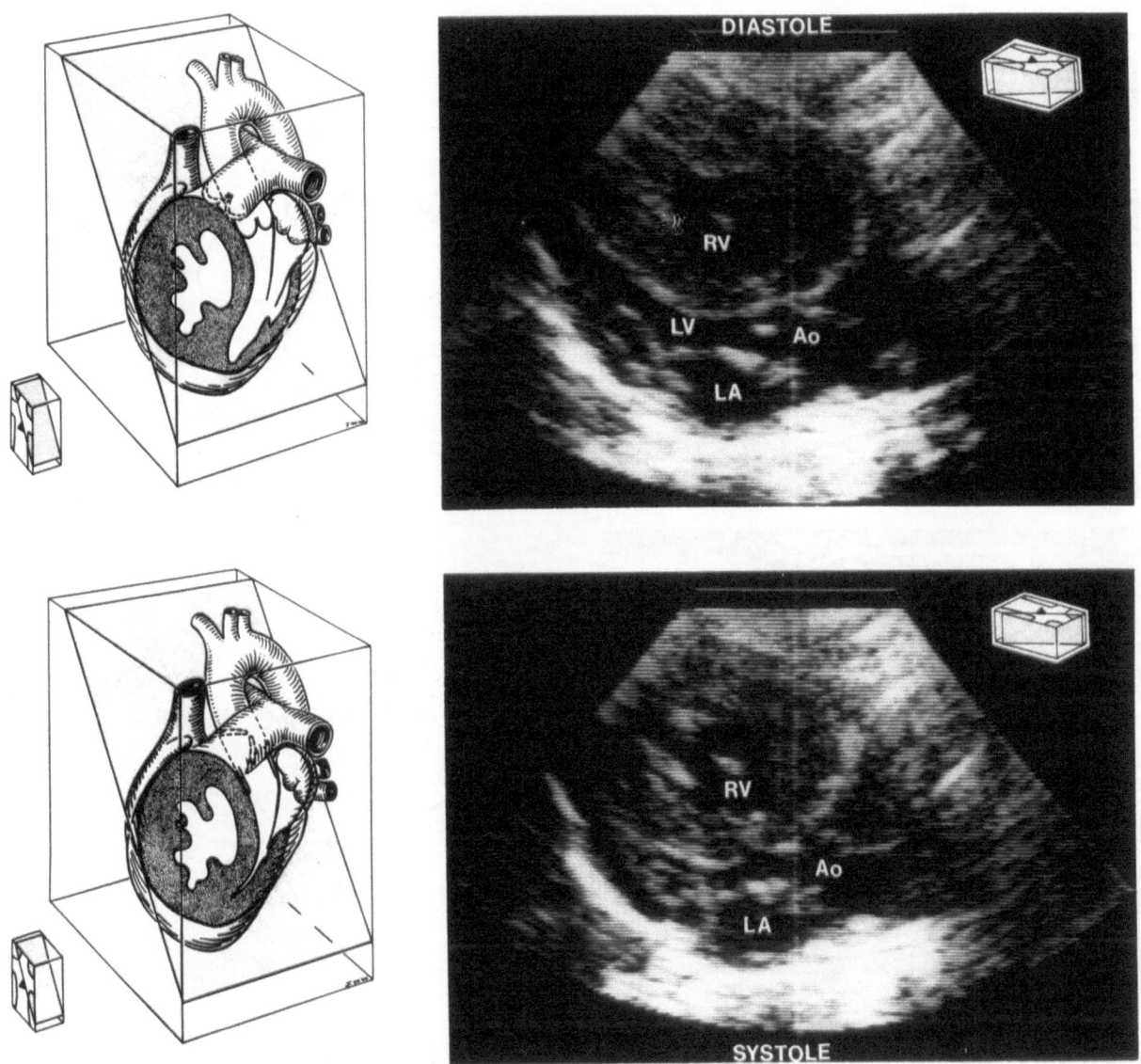

Figure 6.2. Parasternal long axis views of the same patient as in Figure 6.1 showing the spherical and grossly hypertrophic right ventricle. The left ventricle is flattened and its cavity is obliterated during systole.

RV = right ventricle, LV = left ventricle, LA = left atrium, Ao = aorta.

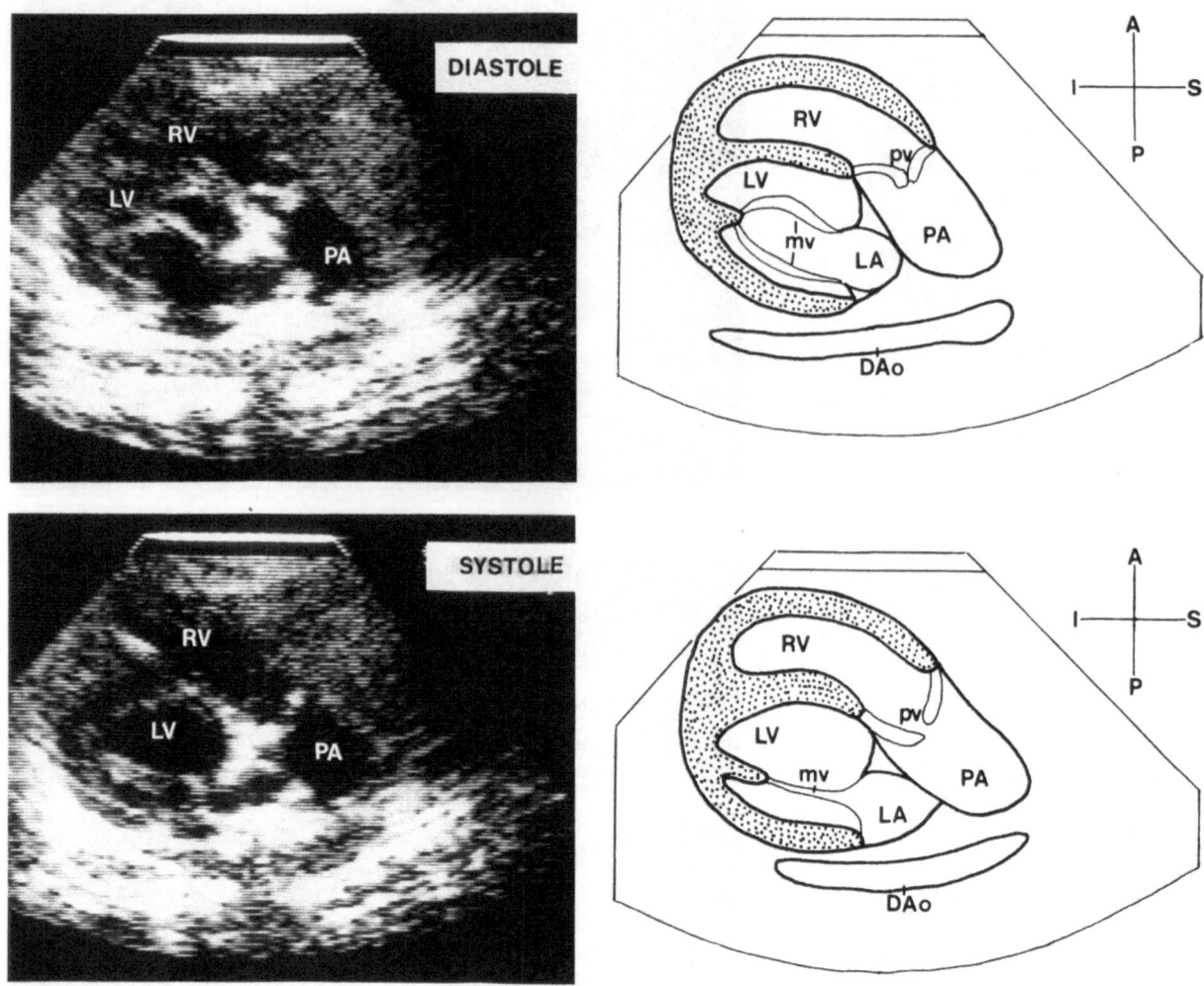

Figure 6.3. Parasternal sagittal two-dimensional echocardiogram of a patient with marked pulmonary valve stenosis. In diastole the thickened pulmonary valve is closed and the mitral valve is open. During systole the pulmonary valve shows the typical doming pattern.

RV = right ventricle, LV = left ventricle, mv = mitral valve, pv = pulmonary valve, LA = left atrium, PA = pulmonary artery, DAo = descending aorta.

7. TETRALOGY OF FALLOT AND TRUNCUS ARTERIOSUS

Fallot's tetralogy consists of the combination of ventricular septal defect, overriding of the aorta, pulmonary stenosis and secondary right ventricular hypertrophy. The pulmonary stenosis is typically an infundibular obstruction consisting of hypertrophic muscle bundles. In addition, there may be a valvular or supravalvular stenosis with or without hypoplasia of the pulmonary valve and main pulmonary artery. Hence, the stenosis is commonly not a localized obstruction but an elongated narrowing along the right ventricular outflow tract and the pulmonary artery.

Clinically, this causes a high-pitched ejection murmur in the left parasternal area. Initially, the systolic murmur may stop just before the second sound. In the absence of cyanosis this may erroneously suggest an isolated ventricular septal defect. However, the electrocardiogram is compatible with right ventricular hypertrophy and the chest X-ray may reveal the 'coeur en sabot' silhouette, diminished pulmonary vascular markings and occasionally a right sided aortic arch. In Fallot's tetralogy the cyanosis often develops gradually with progression of infundibular stenosis which augments the R-L ventricular shunt. At the same time the systolic murmur becomes shortened.

Additional two-dimensional echocardiographic information will reveal the actual pathology (1 – 3). The parasternal long axis view will visualize the overriding of the aorta across the interventricular septum (Figure 7.1). The anterior wall of the aorta with the outlet septum has in this case a markedly anterior position compared with the trabecular septum which has its free edge beneath the posterior cusp of the aortic valve. Thus, the overriding of the aorta across the interventricular septum is associated with a malalignment of the outlet and trabecular septa and the ventricular septal defect in Fallot's tetralogy is typically a malalignment defect which does not close spontaneously. The fibrous continuity between the anterior mitral valve leaflet and the posterior wall of the aorta is normal. The short axis view, at the level of the great arteries, reveals the striking difference between the wide ascending aorta and the slender pulmonary artery (Figure 7.2). This case does not show an obstruction of the right ventricular outflow tract. In the echocardiograms of Figure 7.3 the infundibular stenosis is evident. Real-time imaging sometimes shows obliteration of the right ventricular outflow tract during systole. Resolution problems may be encountered, particularly in older children, because the narrow right ventricular outflow tract is close to the anterior chest wall and thus also in the near field of the ultrasonic beam. If possible, the right ventricular outflow tract should be visualized in a subcostal sagittal view because the interposition of the liver between the heart and the transducer overcomes the problem of the near field imaging. Besides, disturbing reflections of the chest wall are avoided. Details of the pulmonary stenosis are best observed by right ventricular angiography.

The overriding of the aorta is not always obvious in the antero-posterior direction i.e. the long axis view. The anterior overriding may even be minimal in this plane (Figure 7.4). Figure 7.5 displays a subcostal view of the same patient as in Figure 7.4 imaging the plane of the ascending aorta and aortic arch. The overriding of the aorta is striking whereby the interventricular septum is situated beneath the left aortic cusp, as seen in the diastolic still frame. The sagittal cut through the pulmonary artery in this patient has a poor resolution in the near field (Figure 7.6). During real-time imaging the pulmonary valve could clearly be localized. Supravalvularly, a narrowing of the small main pulmonary artery is evident.

82

If the pulmonary valve and main pulmonary artery cannot be visualized pulmonary atresia with ventricular septal defect should be suspected. Failure to recognize the structures may be confusing i.e. either it is not seen or it is not present. If the quality of the images is good, as may generally be expected in full-term infants with normal birth weight, failure to demonstrate the pulmonary valve and main pulmonary artery indicates pulmonary atresia. In newborn infants with low birth weights the diameter of the pulmonary artery may not exceed a few millimeters and may be missed.

Especially in the presence of increased pulmonary vascular markings on the chest X-ray and absence of the pulmonary valve on the echocardiogram truncus arteriosus should be suspected. In these cases there is overriding of the single arterial trunk across the interventricular septum. Figure 7.7 shows an example of a truncus arteriosus Edwards type I (4) in which the main pulmonary artery arises from the truncus. Both the subcostal longitudinal and the parasternal long axis views show an arterial trunk branching as it ascends, indicating the presence of a truncus (5). Other striking features in this example are the hypertrophy of the ventricles and the thickening of the truncal valve.

References

1. Sahn DJ, Terry R, O'Rourke R, Leopold G, Friedman WF: Multiple crystal cross-sectional echocardiography in the diagnosis of cyanotic congenital heart disease. Circulation 50:230 – 238, 1974.
2. Henry WL, Maron BJ, Griffith JM: Cross-sectional echocardiography in the diagnosis of congenital heart disease. Circulation 56:267 – 273, 1977.
3. Caldwell RL, Weyman AE, Hurwitz RA, Girod DA, Feigenbaum H: Right ventricular outflow tract assessment by cross-sectional echocardiography in tetralogy of Fallot. Circulation 59:395 – 402, 1979.
4. Collett RW, Edwards JE: Persistent truncus arteriosus: classification according to anatomic types. Surg Clin North Am 29:1245 – 1270, 1949.
5. Houston AB, Gregory NL, Murtagh E, Coleman EN: Two-dimensional echocardiography in infants with persistent truncus arteriosus. Br Heart J 46:492 – 497, 1981.

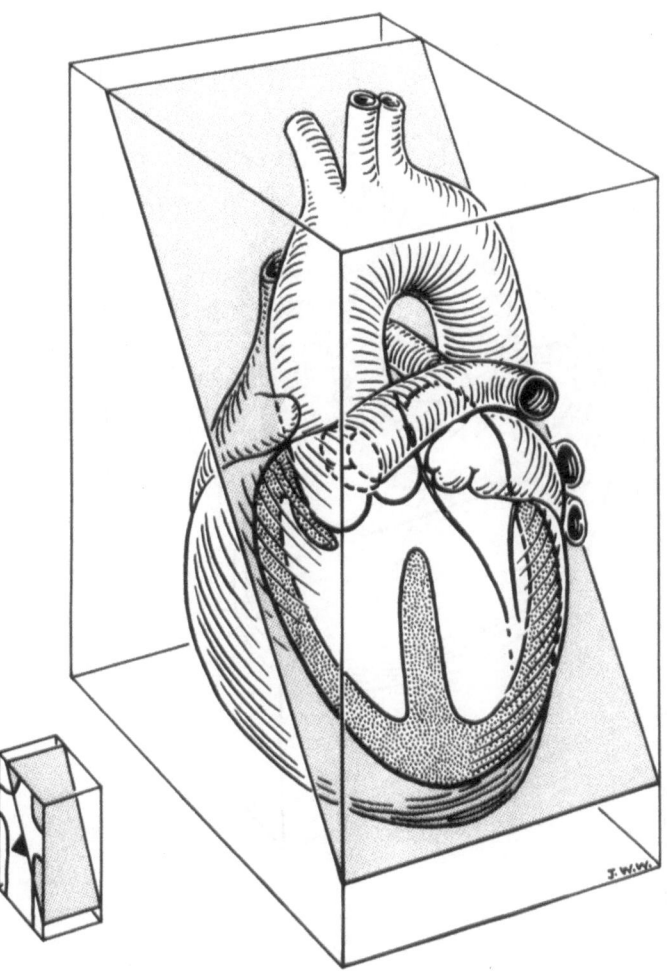

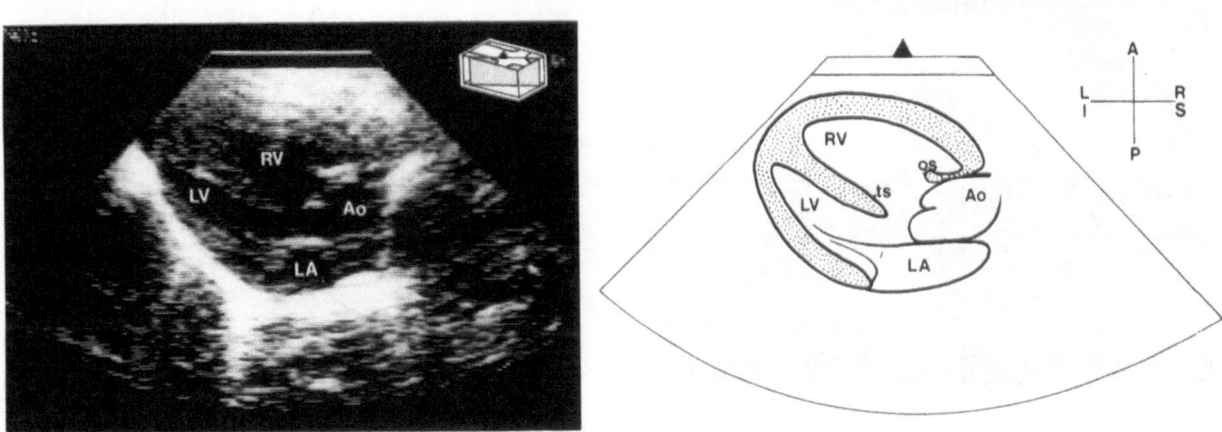

Figure 7.1. Parasternal long axis two-dimensional echocardiogram of a patient with Fallot's tetralogy showing marked overriding of the aorta across the interventricular septum.

LV = *left ventricle*, RV = *right ventricle*, Ao = *aorta*, LA = *left atrium*, ts = *trabecular septum*, os = *outlet septum*.

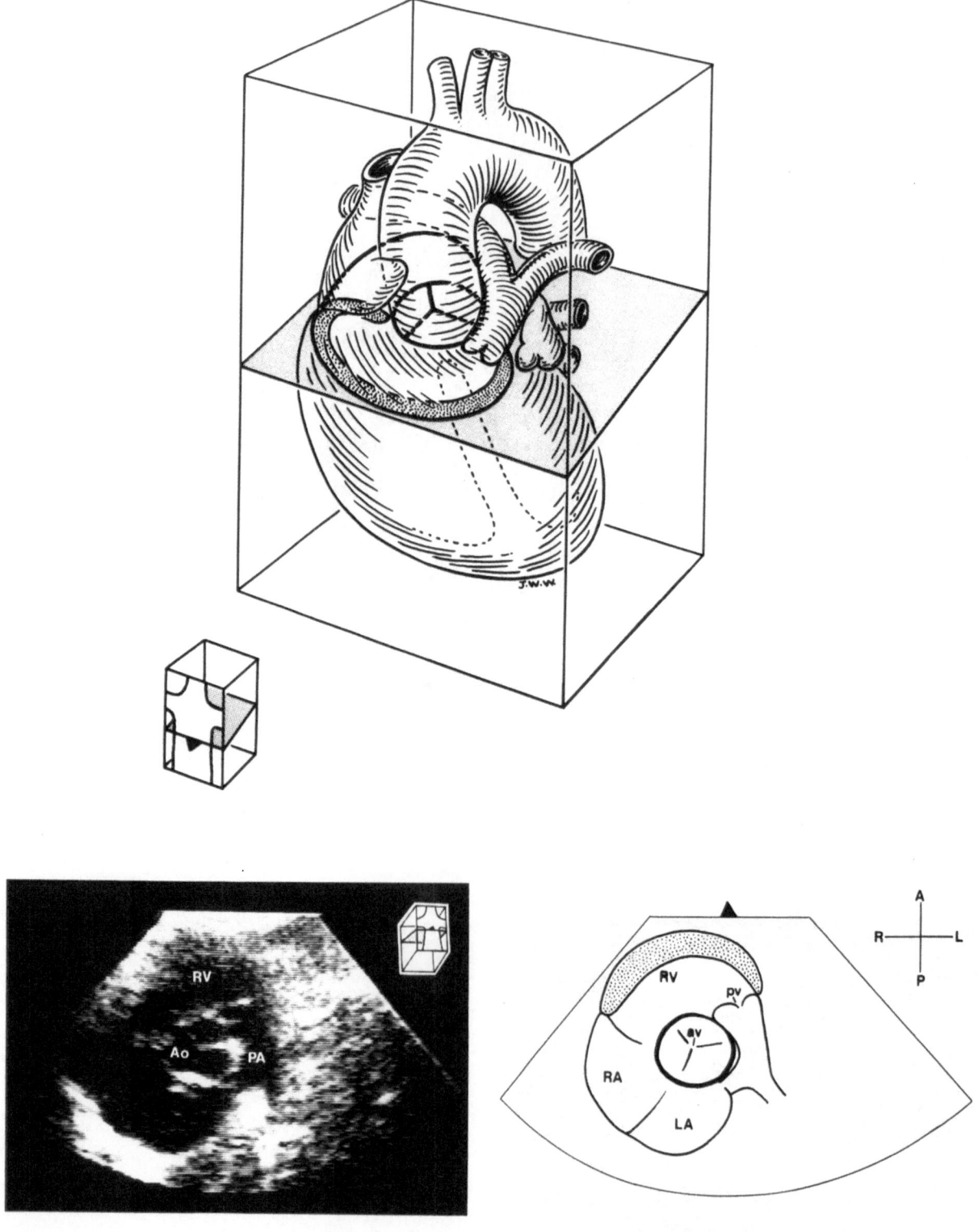

Figure 7.2. Parasternal short axis two-dimensional echocardiogram of a patient with Fallot's tetralogy. Note the small pulmonary artery and the wide aortic valve ring. Infundibular stenosis in the right ventricle is absent.

RV = right ventricle, Ao = aorta, PA = pulmonary artery, RA = right atrium, LA = left atrium, pv = pulmonary valve, av = aortic valve.

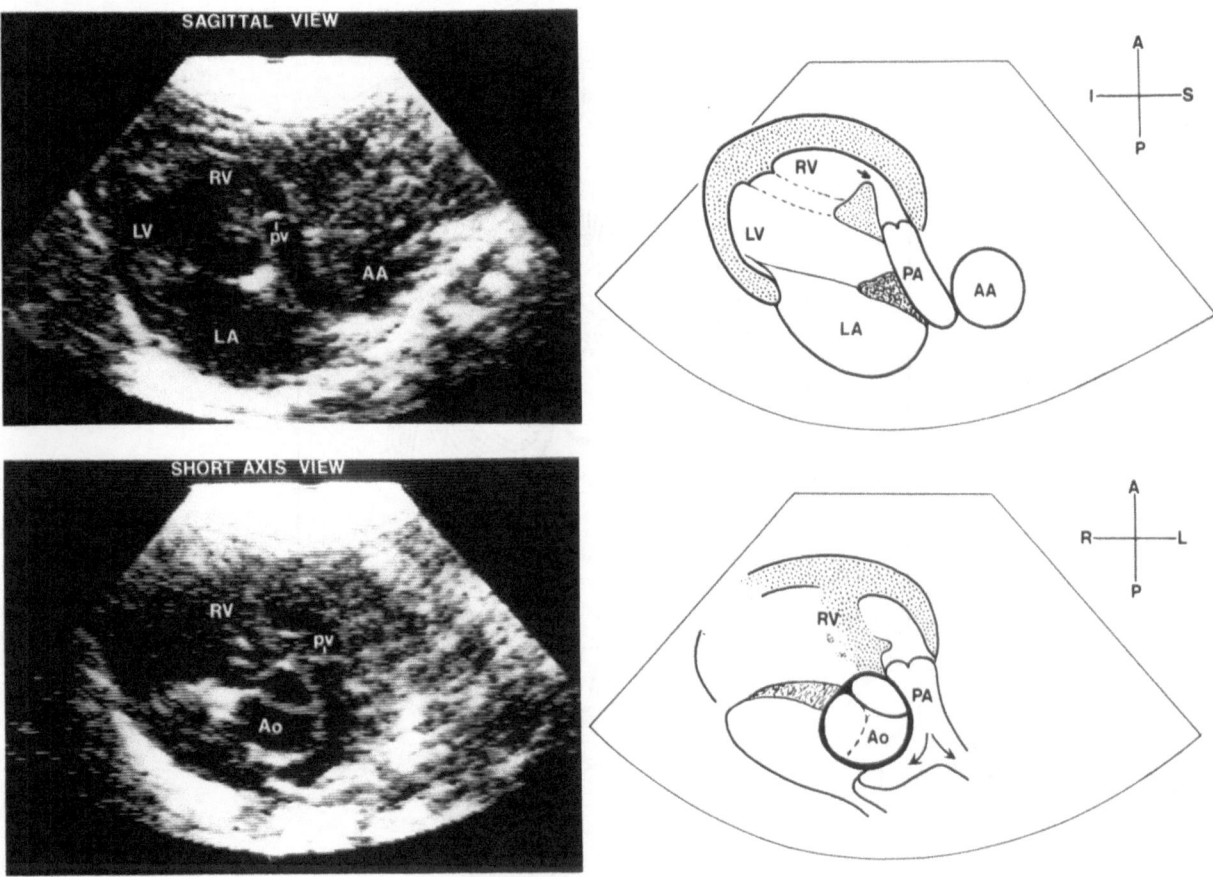

Figure 7.3. Parasternal two-dimensional echocardiograms of patients with tetralogy of Fallot. The pulmonary artery and the pulmonary valve are hypoplastic. In the sagittal view there is narrowing in the subpulmonary region (arrow). The short axis view exhibits a large muscle bundle in the right ventricular outflow tract just anterior to the aorta, dividing the right ventricle into a small outflow part and a much larger inflow part.

RV = right ventricle, LV = left ventricle, PA = pulmonary artery, LA = left atrium, pv = pulmonary valve, AA = aortic arch, Ao = aorta.

86

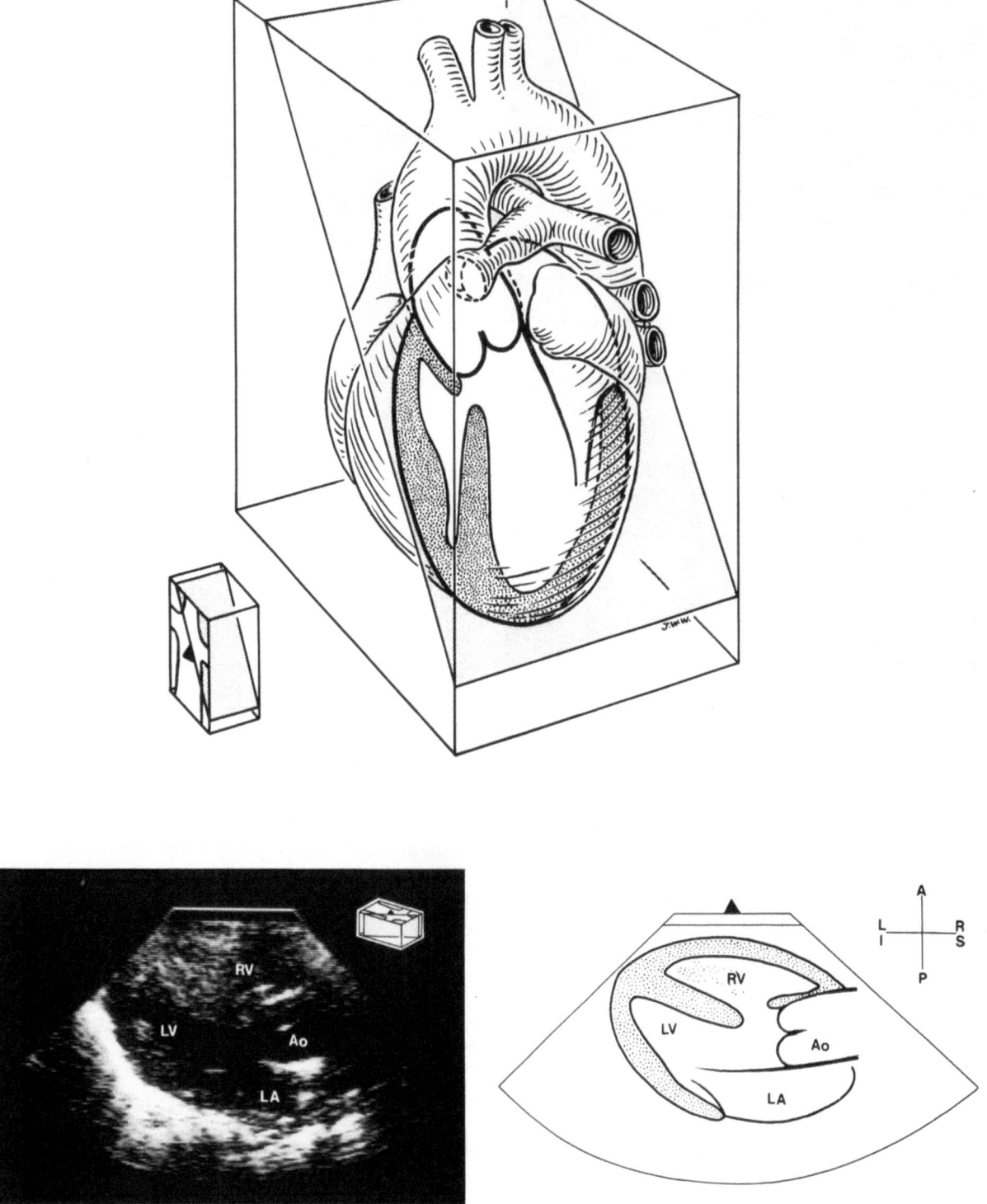

Figure 7.4. Parasternal long axis two-dimensional echocardiogram of a patient with tetralogy of Fallot. The overriding of the aorta across the interventricular septum is minimal and the interventricular communication appears rather small.

LV = left ventricle, RV = right ventricle, Ao = aorta, LA = left atrium.

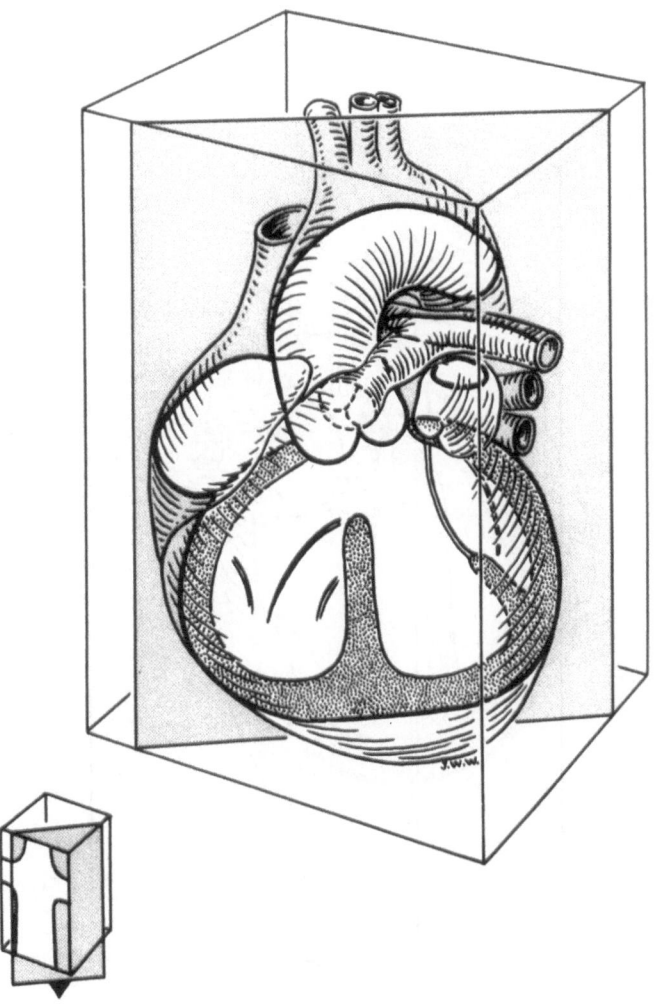

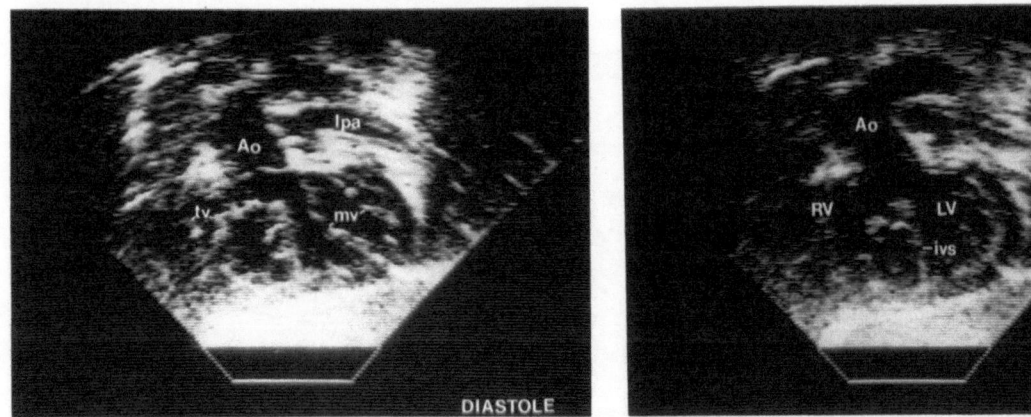

Figure 7.5. Subcostal two-dimensional echocardiogram of the same patient as in Figure 7.4. In this view the overriding of the aorta is obvious and the ventricular septal defect is quite large.

Ao = aorta, tv = tricuspid valve, mv = mitral valve, lpa = left pulmonary artery, RV = right ventricle, LV = left ventricle, ivs = interventricular *septum.*

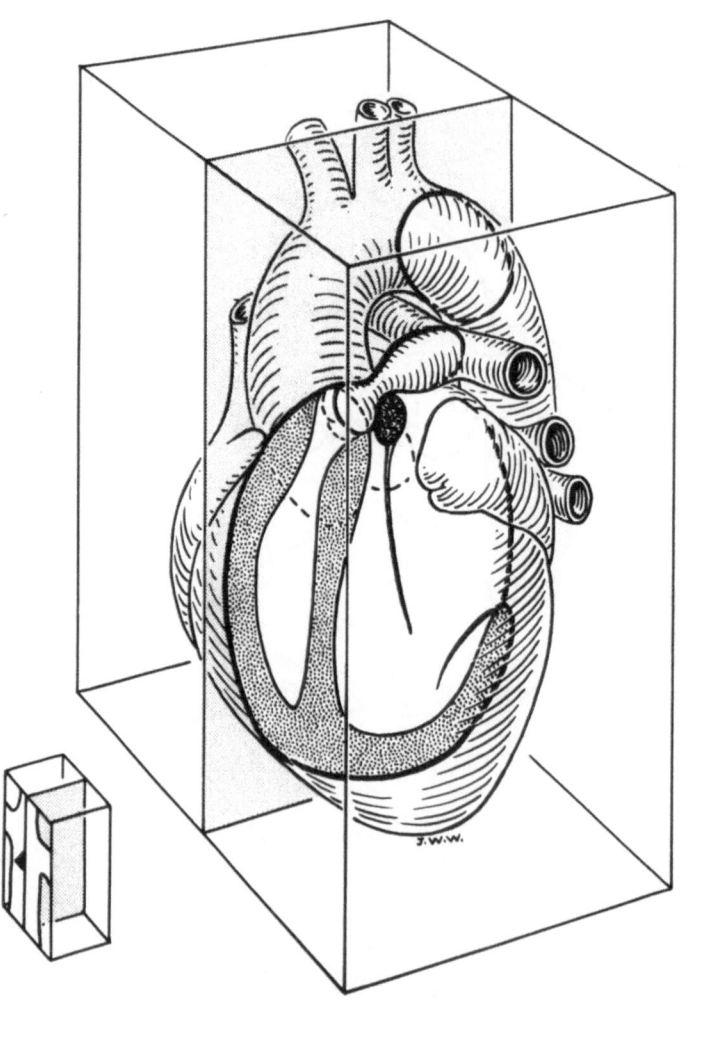

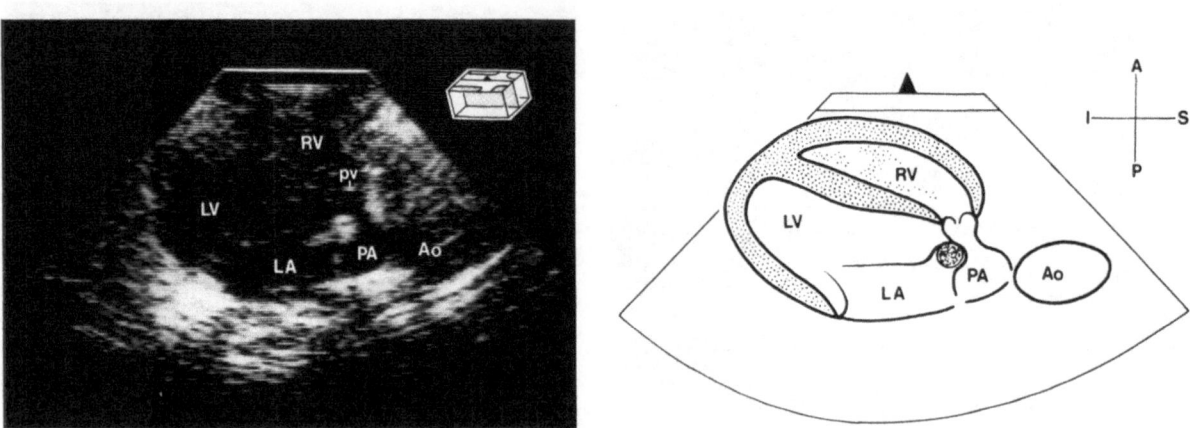

Figure 7.6. Parasternal sagittal view of the same patient as in the two previous figures. There is a localized narrowing of the main pulmonary artery. The pulmonary valve is hypoplastic and the subpulmonary region also seems narrowed.

LV = left ventricle, RV = right ventricle, LA = left atrium, PA = pulmonary artery, Ao = aorta, pv = pulmonary valve.

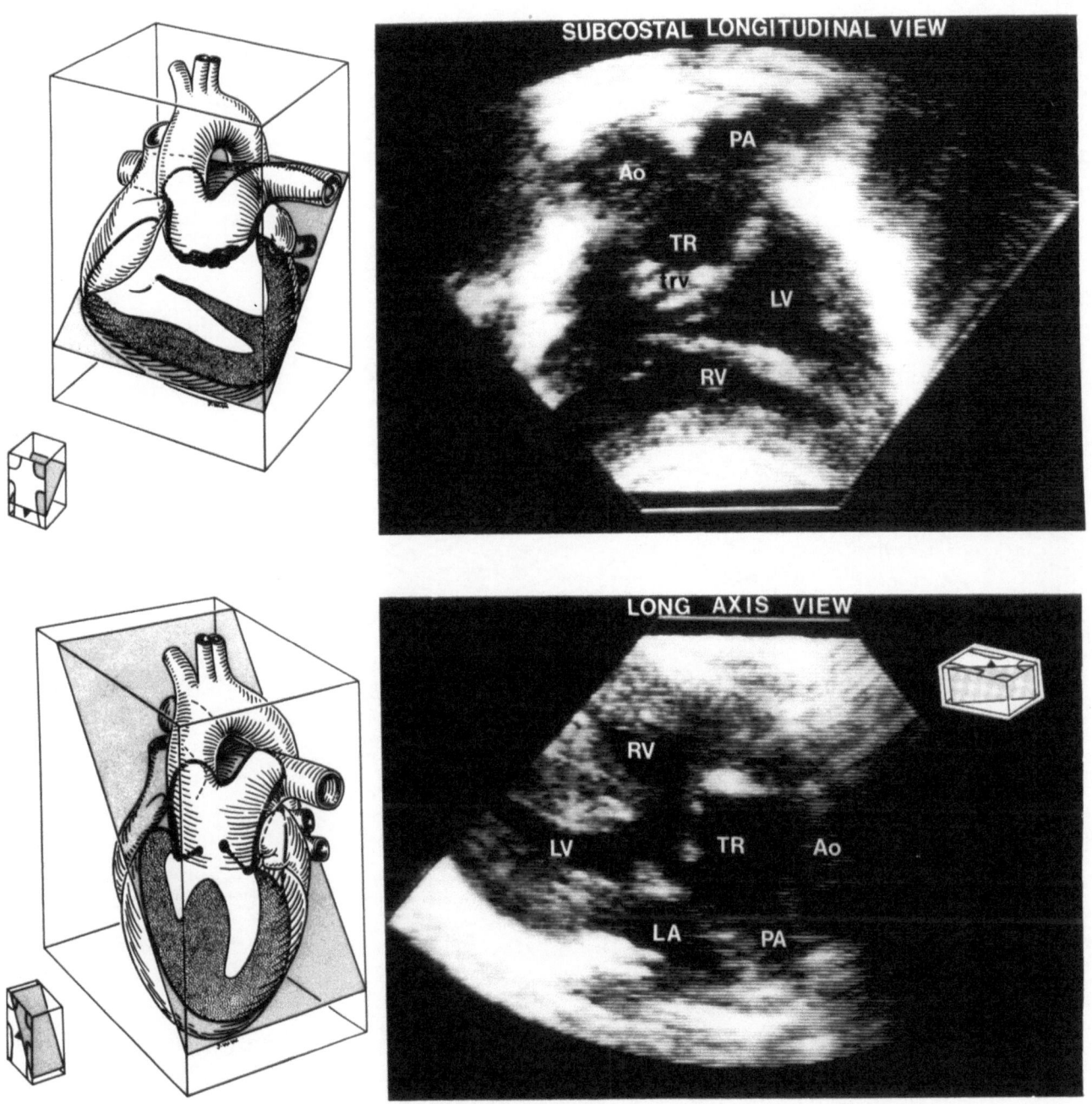

Figure 7.7. Subcostal and parasternal two-dimensional echocardiograms of a patient with truncus arteriosus. The drawing of the subcostal longitudinal view does not show that the actual echocardiographic plane, corresponding with the still frame, was obtained by a slight rotation of the transducer into a right-anterior and left-posterior direction.

Ao = aorta, PA = pulmonary artery, TR = truncus, trv = truncal valve, LV = left ventricle, RV = right ventricle, LA = left atrium.

8. COARCTATION OF THE AORTA

Congestive heart failure in the first weeks of life is frequently caused by coarctation of the aorta, which may be diagnosed by clinical examination. The femoral pulsations are weak or absent with the blood pressure in the arms being considerably higher than in the legs. If the left subclavian artery originates below the level of the coarctation the pressure in the left arm is also low. The electrocardiograms of these infants are compatible with right ventricular hypertrophy or dilatation. The chest X-ray reveals marked cardiomegaly. This corresponds with the severely dilated right ventricle seen by echocardiography. The circulation of blood through the lower part of the body, and thus the kidneys, is reduced, which results in water and salt retention. The left ventricle often has thick walls with a diminished compliance and is frequently slightly smaller than normal. Thus, the fluid retention more readily dilates the right than the left ventricle. The aorta is usually slender and the aortic valve almost always bicuspid (chapter 10). A concomitant mitral lesion, not infrequently seen with coarctation of the aorta (1), e.g. parachute mitral valve, demands careful two-dimensional echocardiographic analysis of the mitral region.

The coarctation is normally situated just distal to the origin of the left subclavian artery. This region can be visualized by two-dimensional echocardiography in the suprasternal view or the parasternal sagittal view of the pulmonary artery and the descending aorta. Sahn, Weyman and Snider and their associates (2, 3, 4) report excellent results in visualizing coarctation of the aorta from the suprasternal notch with two-dimensional echocardiography. In our experience the coarctation may sometimes be clearly displayed but on other occasions the images are vague and suggest a *coarctation* but do not allow accurate assessment of the lesion. Figure 8.1 displays the aortic arch from a schoolgirl with a localized coarctation as seen in the suprasternal view. The left carotid and left subclavian arteries are clearly visible. There appears to be a rather elongated narrowing just distal to the left subclavian artery. Angiocardiography unmistakably revealed a typical localized coarctation. Thus, the drawn-out narrowing, seen on the two-dimensional echocardiogram is an artefact. The suprasternal view seen in Figure 8.2 depicts hypoplasia of the aortic isthmus in an infant with complex congenital heart disease. An additional localized coarctation could not be demonstrated or excluded by echocardiography. Angiocardiography of the aorta showed a localized coarctation besides the hypoplasia. The localized character of the coarctation of another infant is clearly visualized in the parasternal sagittal view of Figure 8.3.

Coarctation or interruption of the aortic arch may be part of a complicated congenital cardiac defect. Equal pressures in both ventricles and a patent ductus distal to the narrowing may mask the presence of the aortic lesion on clinical examination. Besides direct echocardiographic visualisation of the site of the possible narrowing echocontrast studies may be of diagnostic value in some of these cases. In Figure 8.4 interruption of the aorta in a newborn infant with transposition of the great arteries and ventricular septal defect is confirmed by a venous echocontrast study. The two great arteries are visualized in the parasternal sagittal view. The anterior aorta is lying parallel to the posterior main pulmonary artery. In this plane the latter is shown to be continuous through a patent ductus with the descending aorta. A continuation of aortic arch and descending aorta could not be detected suggesting an interruption. Venous echocontrast injection opacifies first the right ventricle

92

and then through the ventricular septal defect contrast enters the left ventricle. On reaching the great arteries the ascending aorta is strongly opacified while the descending aorta shows only a little contrast. During the entire study there was no perceptible difference in opacification between the ascending aorta and the pulmonary artery.

References

1. Rosenquist GC: Congenital mitral valve disease associated with coarctation of the aorta. Circulation 49:985–993, 1974.
2. Sahn DJ, Allen HD, McDonald G, Goldberg SJ: Real-time cross-sectional echocardiographic diagnosis of coarctation of the aorta. Circulation 56:762–769, 1977.
3. Weyman AE, Caldwell RL, Hurwitz RA, Girod DA, Dillon JC, Feigenbaum H, Green D: Cross-sectional echocardiographic detection of aortic obstruction. Circulation 57:498–502, 1978.
4. Snider AR, Silverman NH: Suprasternal notch echocardiography: a two-dimensional technique for evaluating congenital heart disease. Circulation 63:165–173, 1981.

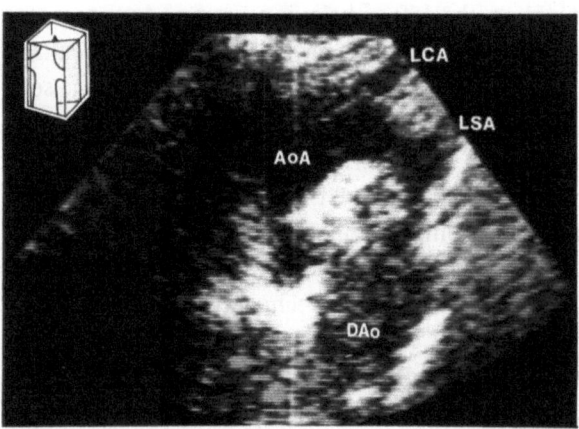
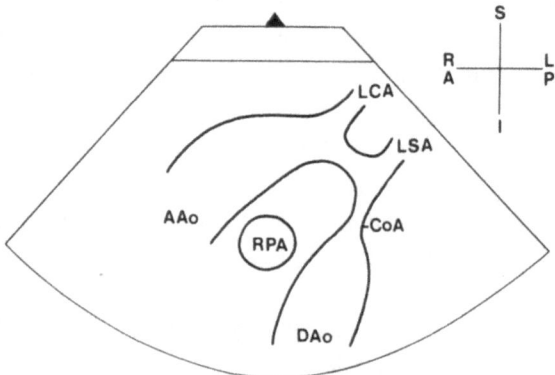

Figure 8.1. Suprasternal two-dimensional echocardiogram of a patient with coarctation of the aorta.

AoA = aortic arch, AAo = ascending aorta, DAo = descending aorta, RPA = right pulmonary artery, LCA = left carotid artery, LSA = left subclavian artery, CoA = coarctation of the aorta.

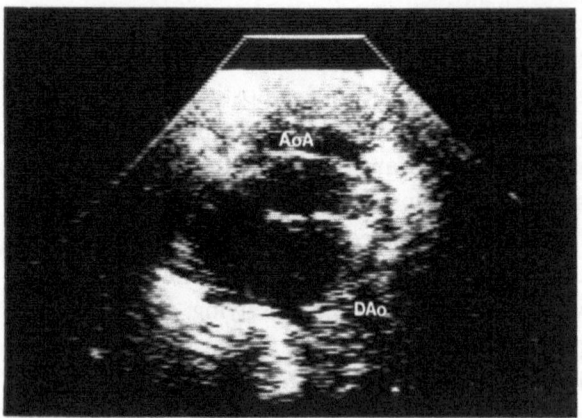
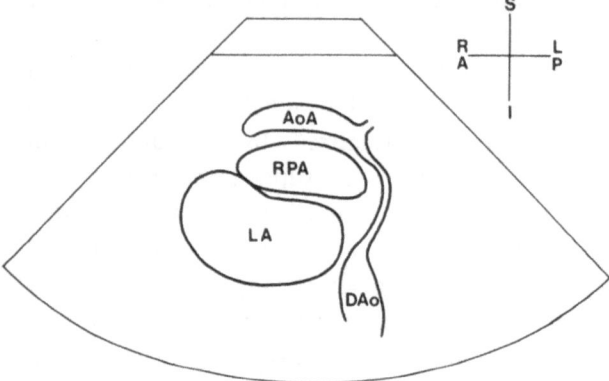

Figure 8.2. Suprasternal two-dimensional echocardiogram in a patient with hypoplasia of the aortic isthmus.

AoA = aortic arch, DAo = descending aorta.

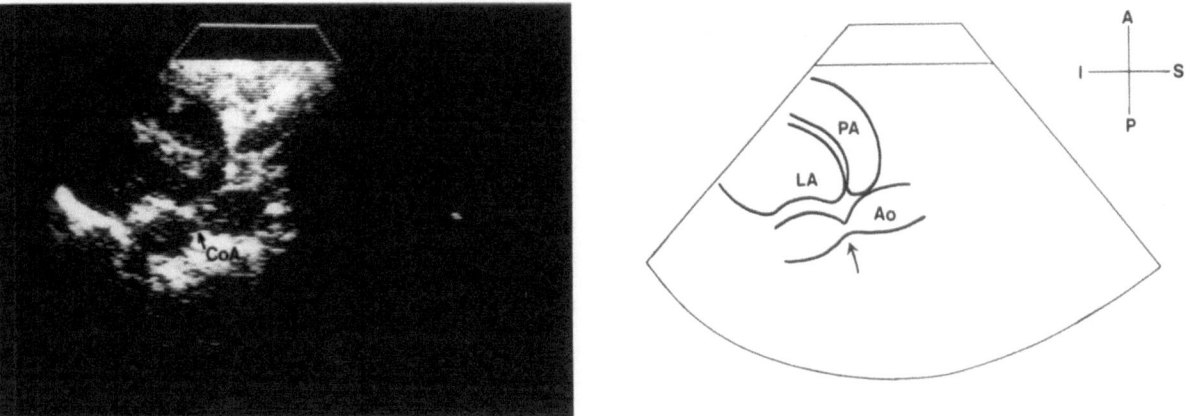

Figure 8.3. Parasternal two-dimensional echocardiogram of a patient with coarctation of the aorta which shows the lesion in a sagittal cross-section through the pulmonary artery and the descending aorta.

LA = left atrium, PA = pulmonary artery, Ao = aorta.

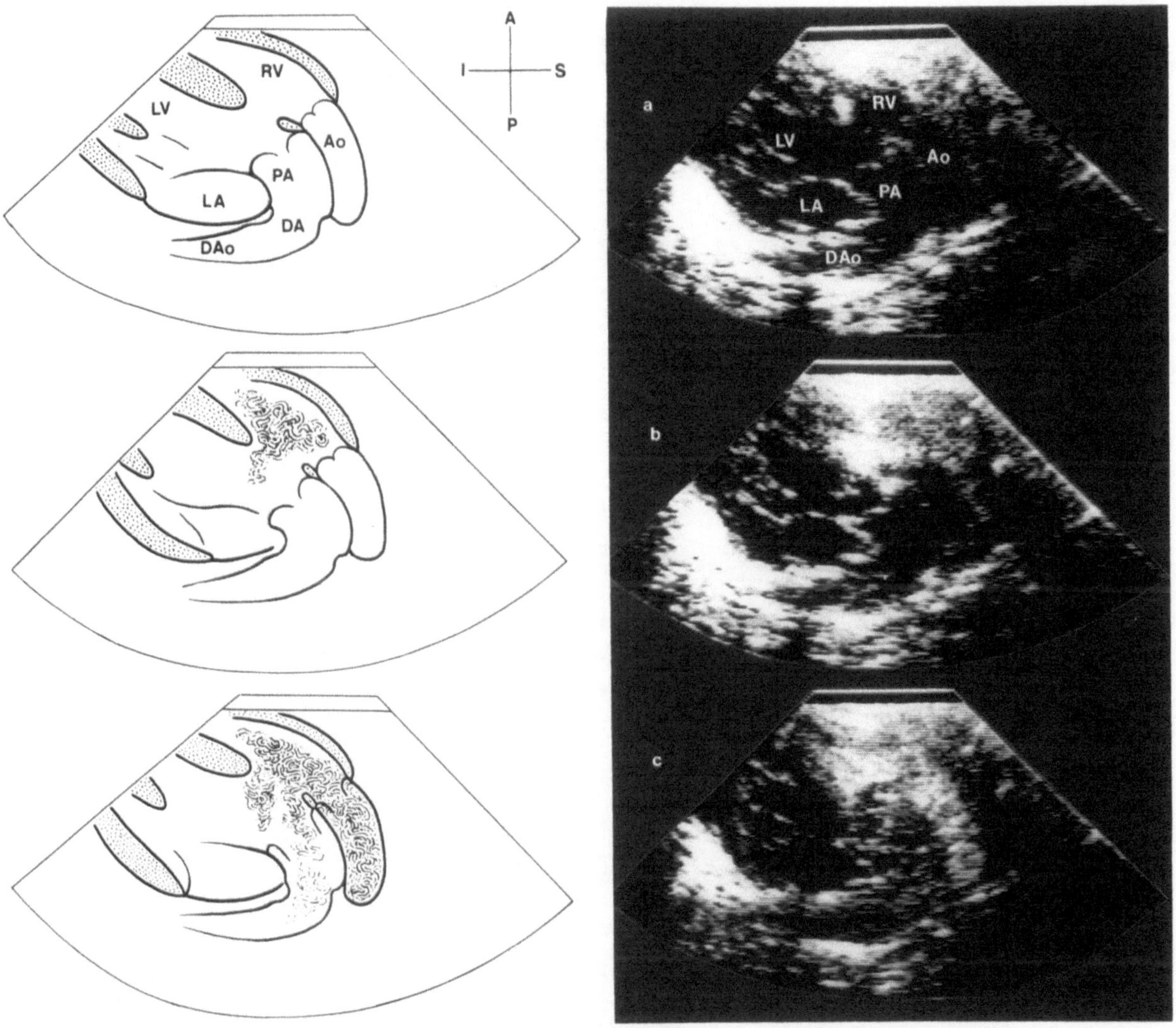

Figure 8.4. Parasternal sagittal two-dimensional echocardiograms of a patient with transposition of the great arteries, interruption of the aorta, ventricular septal defect and persistent ductus arteriosus before (a), and after (b, c) a venous echocontrast injection. The right ventricle is opacified and some echocontrast has passed through the ventricular septal defect (b). When echocontrast has entered the great arteries the ascending aorta is markedly opacified, while the descending aorta shows hardly any contrast (c).

LV = left ventricle, RV = right ventricle, LA = left atrium, PA = pulmonary artery, DA = ductus arteriosus, Ao = aorta, DAo = descending aorta.

9. TRANSPOSITION OF THE GREAT ARTERIES

In transposition of the great arteries the aorta originates from the anatomical right ventricle and the main pulmonary artery from the anatomical left ventricle. The condition is also referred to as d-transposition of the great arteries, or can be described as atrioventricular concordance with ventriculo-arterial discordance. The aorta is usually situated to the right and anterior, or to the right and lateral of the main pulmonary artery. The aorta may also be positioned directly anterior to the main pulmonary artery. Rarely the position of the aorta may be posterior and to the right, or anterior and to the left of the main pulmonary artery (1, 2). The right branch of the pulmonary artery always passes beneath the aortic arch.

Transposition of the great arteries occurs as an 'isolated' anomaly but it is often associated with a ventricular septal defect and/or persistent ductus arteriosus. Occasionally it is seen in combination with left ventricular outflow tract obstruction and/or pulmonary stenosis.

Transposition of the great arteries with intact interventricular septum

Transposition of the great arteries with intact interventricular septum should be suspected when a newborn infant shows increasing cyanosis from birth without clinical evidence of pulmonary, cerebral or haemopoetic disturbances to account for the cyanosis. There are no respiratory difficulties and there is no cardiac murmur. The electrocardiogram is compatible with normal physiological right ventricular preponderance. The chest X-ray may show a heart with typical egg-like appearance and the pulmonary vascular markings are usually increased. Administration of 100% oxygen hardly influences the low oxygen concentration of the blood.

The condition can accurately be diagnosed by two-dimensional echocardiography (3, 4, 5). The ventriculo-arterial discordance can be demonstrated in the parasternal and subcostal views. A parasternal long axis view of an infant with transposition of the great arteries is shown in Figure 9.1. Two striking features are demonstrated. Firstly, the two semilunar valves are simultaneously visualized. The anterior semilunar valve is situated more superiorly and, depending on the plane of cross-section, more to the right than the posterior valve. This relationship is typical for d-transposition of the great arteries. The second feature is the backward sweep of the posterior great artery just distal to its valve (6). As such the inferior wall of the posterior artery comprises the roof of the left atrium. This backward sweep identifies that artery as the main pulmonary artery. The aorta is recognized by the straight, cranial and retrosternal course of the ascending aorta before it continues into the aortic arch superior to the pulmonary artery (3).

Another feature typical of d-transposition of the great arteries is the initial parallel relationship of the two great arteries. This is not evident in Figure 9.1, because the walls of the aorta are not adequately visualized. However, it is clearly demonstrated in another case with an almost complete antero-posterior relationship of the great arteries (Figure 9.2). The parasternal short axis view also shows the parallelism of the great arteries. In transverse cross-section they are visualized as two adjacent circles (3, 4). In the presence of normally related great arteries this cross-section shows the sausage-shaped shadow of the right ventricular outflow tract and the main pulmonary artery lying anterior to the circular shadow of the transversely cut ascending aorta. The parasternal view shown in Figure 9.3 was ob-

96

tained by a slight cranial angulation of the ultra-sonic beam which visualized the bifurcation of the posterior artery. This bifurcation identifies that artery as the pulmonary artery (6). In d-transposition of the great arteries the bifurcation of the posteriorly situated pulmonary artery can usually be visualized in the subcostal longitudinal view (5) (Figure 9.4). In this few months' old infant the right ventricle is dilated. The interventricular septum is convex to the left and flattens the left ventricle. This produces an angle between the long axis of the left ventricle and the axis of the main pulmonary artery. Therefore, it can be difficult to demonstrate the left ventricle and the main pulmonary artery simultaneously in a parasternal long axis view.

Flattening of the left ventricle develops as early as in the first week of life when the pressure in the left ventricle diminishes because of the decreasing pulmonary vascular resistance. The high systemic pressure in the right ventricle causing leftward bulging of the interventricular septum which reduces the normal egg-like left ventricle to a pancake-like structure.

The subcostal longitudinal view and subcostal frontal view of a patient with transposition of the great arteries are shown in Figure 9.5 and 9.6. These views clearly demonstrate that the aorta originates from the right ventricle. In the longitudinal view the posterior great artery arises from the left ventricle. Superior to the posterior great artery a large almost horizontally traversing space is visible. When the ultrasonic beam is directed more frontally this space appears to be continuous with the anterior great artery which originates from the right ventricle. This artery has initially a straight, cranial and retrosternal course whereafter it arches across the posterior great artery. This identifies the artery as the ascending aorta with the aortic arch. The anterior ventricle can be distinguished as the right ventricle by the irregular endocardial surface, caused by the marked trabeculae, and the apically inserted papillary muscle. The posterior left ventricle has a smooth wall.

Recently, the anatomical correction of transposition of the great arteries (the arterial Switch operation) has been reintroduced as a possible alternative of the physiological corrections of Mustard and Senning. In order to switch the great

arteries successfully the left ventricle must be able to maintain the circulation against the systemic vascular resistance. As a normal physiological response to the reduction of the pulmonary vascular resistance the pressure in the left ventricle diminishes after birth. Because of this the increase of wall thickness in the left ventricle will be markedly retarded in the first year of life compared with the normal heart. If anatomical correction is intended the pressure in the left ventricle may be augmented by a constriction i.e. banding of the main pulmonary artery in order to provoke development of the left ventricular walls. Sometimes this is combined with an aorto-pulmonary shunt to establish an optimal left ventricular volume load. Thus the left ventricle may be prepared for an anatomical correction at a later stage.

Figure 9.7 displays a short axis view of a patient with transposition of the great arteries showing the typical pancaked cavity of the left ventricle.

Figure 9.8 exhibits the long and short axis views of a three months' old patient with transposition of the great arteries after tight banding of the pulmonary artery. The thickness of the wall of the left ventricle is almost the same as that of the right ventricle. The short axis view shows the globular shape of the left ventricle as a result of the suprasystemic pressure.

The effect of the combination of the main pulmonary artery banding and the aorto-pulmonary shunt in the patient with transposition of the great arteries is exhibited echocardiographically in Figure 9.9. The interventricular septum is slightly convex to the left in end-systole which means that the left ventricular pressure is not beyond that in the right ventricle. The left ventricular volume and wall thickness insinuate a successful preparatory operation for an anatomical correction.

The two-dimensional echocardiograms of a patient after an arterial switch operation is demonstrated in Figure 9.10.

The postoperative echocardiograms of a patient with a Mustard correction are shown in Figure 9.11 and 9.12.

In the Mustard operation the atrial septum is exchanged for a baffle that tunnels the superior vena cava via the 'roof' and inferior vena cava via the 'floor' of the atrial cavity to the mitral orifice. The original left atrium is continuous with the remainder of the right atrium at the angle of the superior and inferior caval tunnels. At this site the pulmonary venous blood flows below the superior and over the inferior tunnel towards the tricuspid orifice. The inferior tunnel can be visualized in the parasternal four chamber view. When the ultrasonic beam is directed cranially the connection between the left atrium and right atrium can be seen. The superior tunnel can be visualized when the plane of the echo-beam is directed from the parasternal long axis view to the right. The suprasternal and subcostal windows can also successfully be used (7).

Transposition of the great arteries with ventricular septal defect

The haemodynamics and the clinical course of events in transposition of the great arteries and ventricular septal defect depend on the size of the ventricular septal defect. The ventricular septal defect is often large giving rise to equal or almost equal pressures in both ventricles. Physiological diminution of the pulmonary vascular resistance after birth markedly augments the pulmonary flow with volume overload of the left heart. This may induce cardiac failure with or without pulmonary oedema. These patients present early in life. Immediate palliative treatment may consist of a balloon septostomy to alleviate the extremely elevated left atrial volume and pressure overload. Unless a corrective operation is contemplated early in life banding of the main pulmonary artery may be carried out to prevent cardiac failure and pulmonary vascular disease. The remaining volume overload and elevated afterload stimulate adequate development of the left ventricle. This leaves the choice of type of corrective procedure open to a later stage.

In the absence of cardiac failure recognition of the anomaly may be delayed. Because of the augmented pulmonary blood flow cyanosis may be mild or absent which may lead to the erroneous diagnosis of isolated ventricular septal defect.

As pulmonary vascular disease may be an early complication, prompt diagnosis and treatment is important.

Transposition of the great arteries and ventricular septal defect should always be suspected in the presence of mild cyanosis, a blowing high-pitched pan- or decrescendo systolic murmur, a single second sound, pulmonary plethora and biventricular hypertrophy. If the ventricular septal defect is small spontaneous closure may occur and the clinical course is like that of transposition of the great arteries with intact interventricular septum with marked cyanosis.

Ventricular septal defects in the presence of transposition of the great arteries are of two types, the 'normal' ventricular septal defects as described in chapter 2 and the malalignment defects. In the latter the defect divides the interventricular septum in such a way that parts of it are no longer aligned.

Figure 9.13 shows the subcostal longitudinal view of a patient with transposition of the great arteries and a perimembranous ventricular septal defect. The defect is situated immediately below the pulmonary valve, which location on the right side corresponds with the level of the attachment of the septal leaflet of the tricuspid valve. There is no malalignment which was confirmed by several other views. Early banding of the main pulmonary artery was performed because of severe cardiac failure. The site of the band and the degree of narrowing can be observed in the subcostal view. Perimembranous defects are frequently seen with transposition of the great arteries. Pure muscular inlet defects seldom occur. Defects in the trabecular septum were usually too small for direct echocardiographic visualization. They may be localized by venous echocontrast injections whereby the smaller R-L atrial shunt does not mask the larger R-L ventricular shunt.

Figure 9.14 and 9.15 display the parasternal and subcostal echocardiograms of a patient with transposition of the great arteries and ventricular septal defect with the great arteries in a side by side relationship. The subcostal view clearly shows the defect. There is no sign of malalignment. However, in the long axis view the right ventricle appears to be extended anterior to the outflow area of the left ventricle and the defect spreads into the anterior part of the interventricular septum. Slight overriding of the pulmonary artery across the septum is seen and indicates a malalignment of the outlet- and trabecular parts of the septum. In this patient the malalignment was the probable cause of a serious complication after the arterial switch

98

operation. Subsequent to closure of the ventricular septal defect and retransposition of the great arteries severe subaortic stenosis was observed. Apparently, closure of the ventricular septal defect in this case had markedly reduced the outflow area of the left ventricle. A more striking example of malalignment of the outlet- and trabecular parts of the septum in a patient with transposition of the great arteries is shown in Figure 9.16. The overriding of the main pulmonary artery across the interventricular septum is evident in the subcostal longitudinal view. The subcostal sagittal and frontal views show simultaneously the malaligned outlet- and trabecular septa. In the former view the outlet septum is seen as a continuation of the aorto- pulmonary septum. Compared with the location of the trabecular septum, the outlet septum is displaced anteriorly and to the right. Another feature in the subcostal frontal view is the subaortic narrowing of the right ventricular outflow tract by a muscle bundle on the right and the outlet septum on the left. Cardiac catheterisation, before closure of the ventricular septal defect and retransposition of the great arteries, did not reveal a systolic pressure gradient across the right ventricular outflow tract. Postoperatively a marked gradient was manifest necessitating a patch across the right ventricular outflow tract. Another feature to be mentioned is the abnormality of the tricuspid valve shown in the subcostal sagittal view. The septal part of this valve clearly is inserted into the trabecular septum at the crest of the ventricular septal defect.

Transposition of the great arteries, ventricular septal defect and left ventricular outflow septal tract obstruction

Patients with transposition of the great arteries, ventricular septal defect and left ventricular outflow tract obstruction and/or pulmonary stenosis usually present with cyanosis in the first months of life. They have a loud harsh systolic murmur. The pulmonary circulation is restricted, therefore cardiac failure does not occur. Instead, if the left ventricular outflow tract obstruction is severe, there is marked pulmonary hypoperfusion and the patient is severely cyanotic early in life.

The outflow tract obstruction may be valvular or subvalvular. Sometimes the entire pulmonary vascular system is hypoplastic.

Figure 9.17 and 9.18 display the two-dimensional echocardiograms of a patient who received an aorto-pulmonary shunt because of severe pulmonary hypoperfusion. The subcostal frontal view reveals a wide aorta which clearly communicates with the right ventricle. The subcostal longitudinal view visualizes the hypoplastic main pulmonary artery. There was no echocardiographic communication between main pulmonary artery and the ventricular space. Pulmonary valve movements were absent. At the origin of the main pulmonary artery there are multiple echo's. This is seen in the subcostal longitudinal and the parasternal long axis views. There was no obvious malalignment of parts of the interventricular septum. The defect was of the perimembranous type.

A rare type of left ventricular outflow tract obstruction in transposition of the great arteries with intact interventricular septum and persistent ductus arteriosus is described in chapter 5.

References

1. Marin-Garcia J, Edwards JE: Atypical d-transposition of the great arteries: anterior pulmonary trunk. Am J Cardiol 46:507 – 510, 1980.
2. Bass NM, Roche AHG, Brandt PWT, Neutze JM: Echocardiography in assessment of infants with complete d-transposition of the great arteries. Br Heart J 40:1165 – 1173, 1978.
3. Sahn DJ, Ferry R, O'Rourke R, Leopold G, Friedman WF: Multiple crystal cross-sectional echocardiography in the diagnosis of cyanotic congenital heart disease. Circulation 50:230 – 238, 1974.
4. Henry WL, Maron BJ, Griffith JM, Redwood DR, Ebstein SE: Differential diagnosis of anomalies of the great arteries by real-time two-dimensional echocardiography. Circulation 51:283 – 291, 1975.
5. Bierman FZ, Williams RG: Prospective diagnosis of d-transposition of the great arteries in neonates by subxiphoid two-dimensional echocardiography. Circulation 60:1496 – 1502, 1979.
6. Houston AB, Gregory NL, Coleman EN: Echocardiographic identification of aorta and main pulmonary artery in complete transposition. Br Heart J 40:377 – 382, 1978.
7. Aziz KU, Paul MH, Bharati S, Cole RB, Muster AJ, Lev M, Idriss FS: Two-dimensional echocardiographic evaluation of Mustard operation for d-transposition of the great arteries. Am J Cardiol 47:654 – 664, 1981.

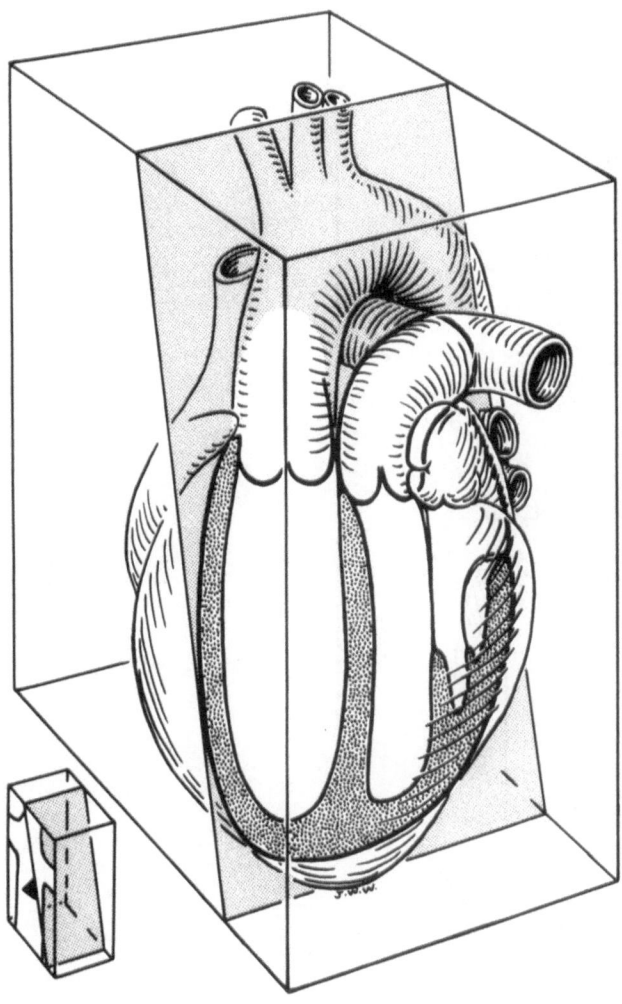

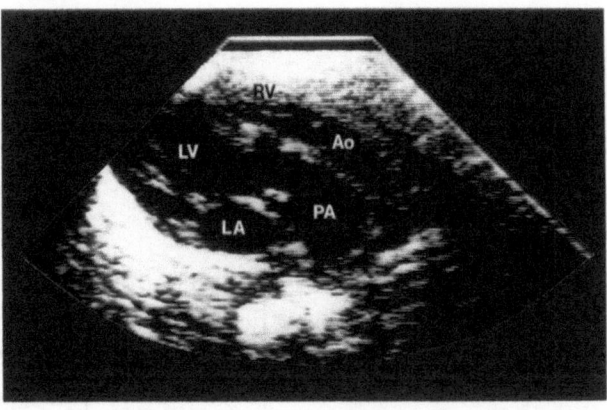

Figure 9.2. Long axis view of a patient with transposition of the great arteries and a direct antero-posterior relationship of the great arteries.

LV = left ventricle, LA = left atrium, RV = right ventricle, Ao = aorta, PA = pulmonary artery.

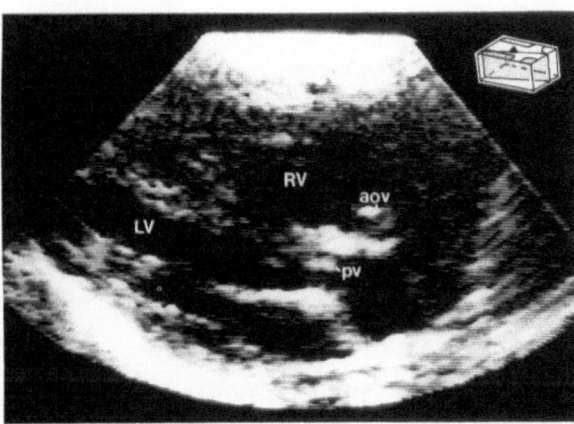

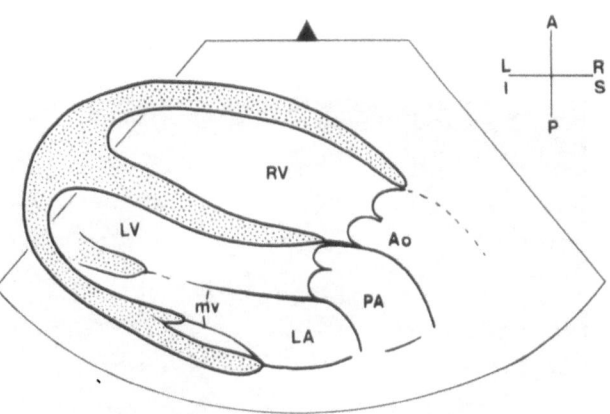

Figure 9.1. Parasternal long axis two-dimensional echocardiogram of a patient with transposition of the great arteries. The two semilunar valves are visualized simultaneously and the posterior arching of the pulmonary artery is evident.

LV = left ventricle, mv = mitral valve, RV = right ventricle, LA = left atrium, PA = pulmonary artery, Ao = aorta.

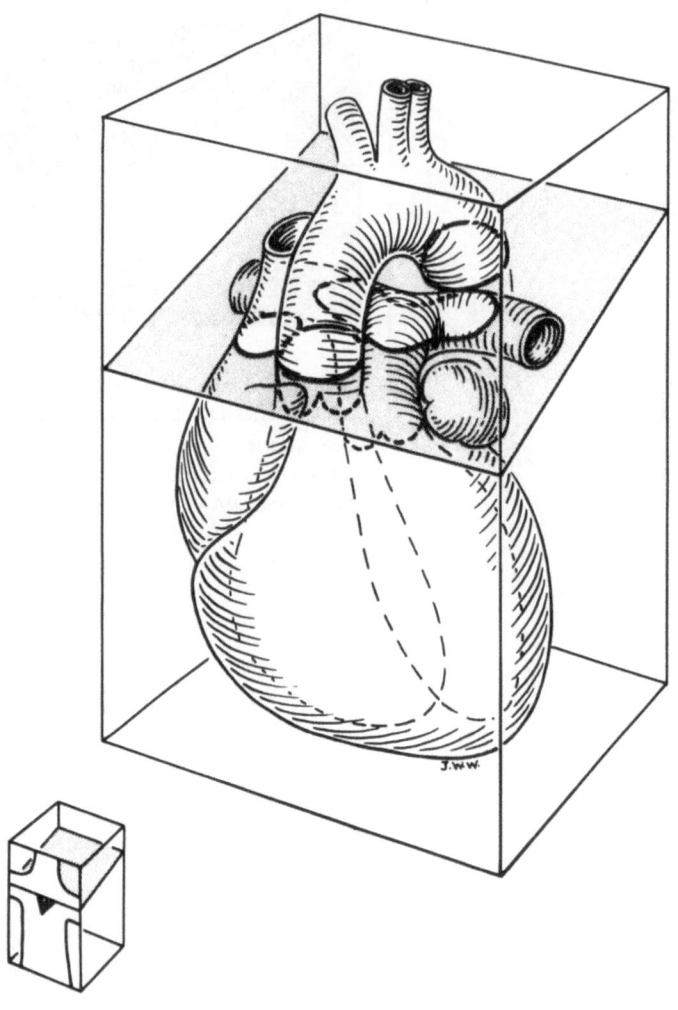

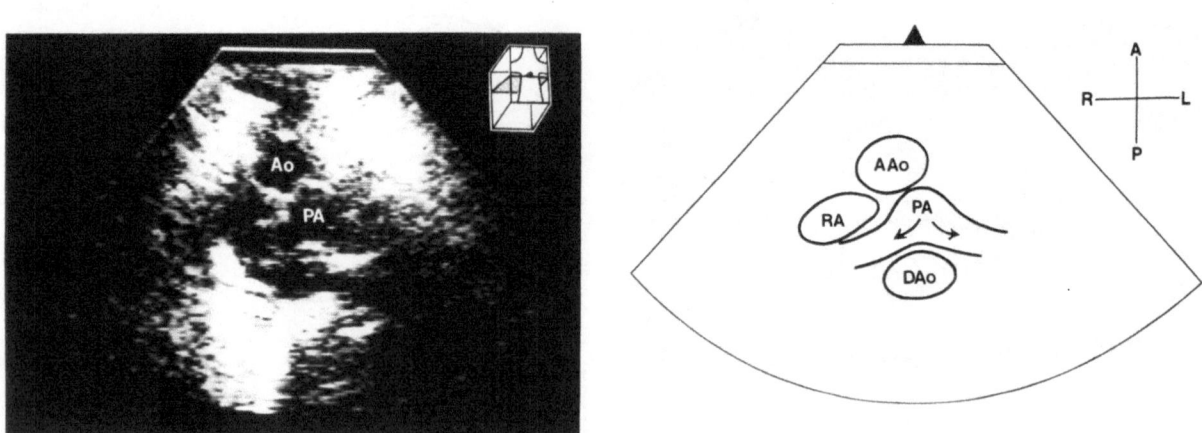

Figure 9.3. Parasternal short axis two-dimensional echocardiogram of a patient with transposition of the great arteries. The posterior great artery bifurcates (arrows).

AAo = ascending aorta, DAo = descending aorta, Ao = aorta, PA = pulmonary artery, RA = right atrium.

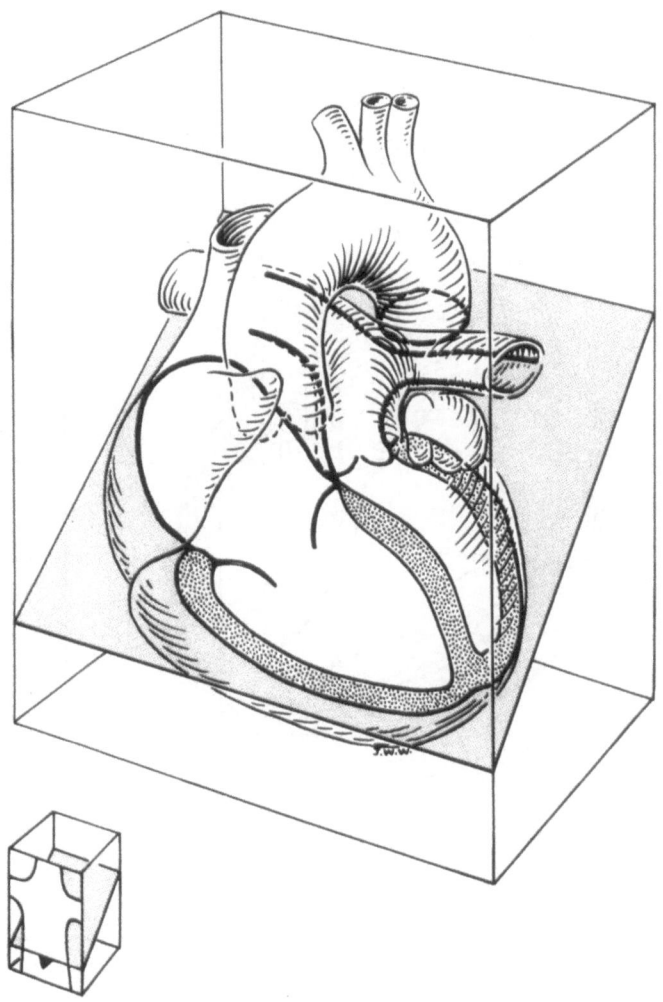

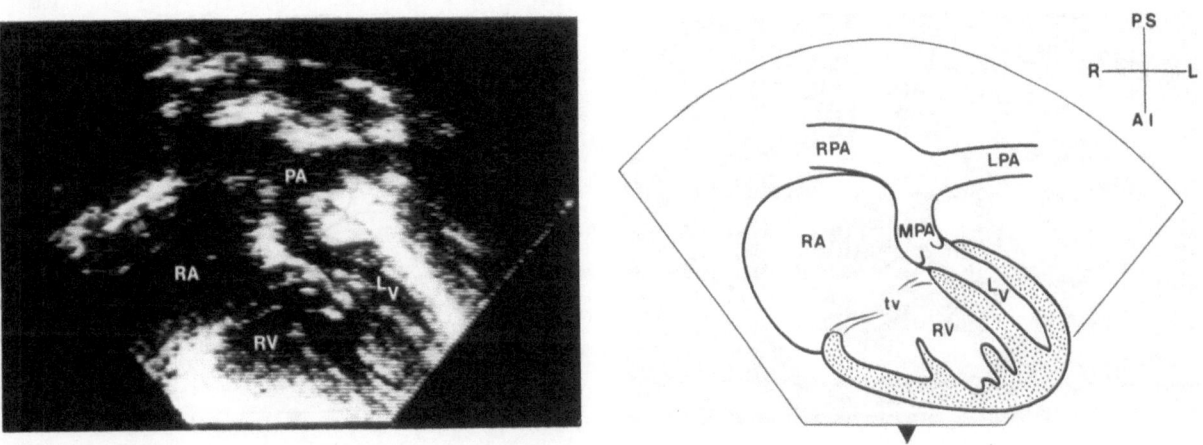

Figure 9.4. Subcostal longitudinal two-dimensional echocardiogram of a patient with transposition of the great arteries. The pulmonary artery originates from a flattened left ventricle. Its bifurcation is clearly shown.

RA = right atrium, tv = tricuspid valve, RV = right ventricle, LV = left ventricle, PA = pulmonary artery, MPA = main pulmonary artery, RPA = right pulmonary artery, LPA = left pulmonary artery.

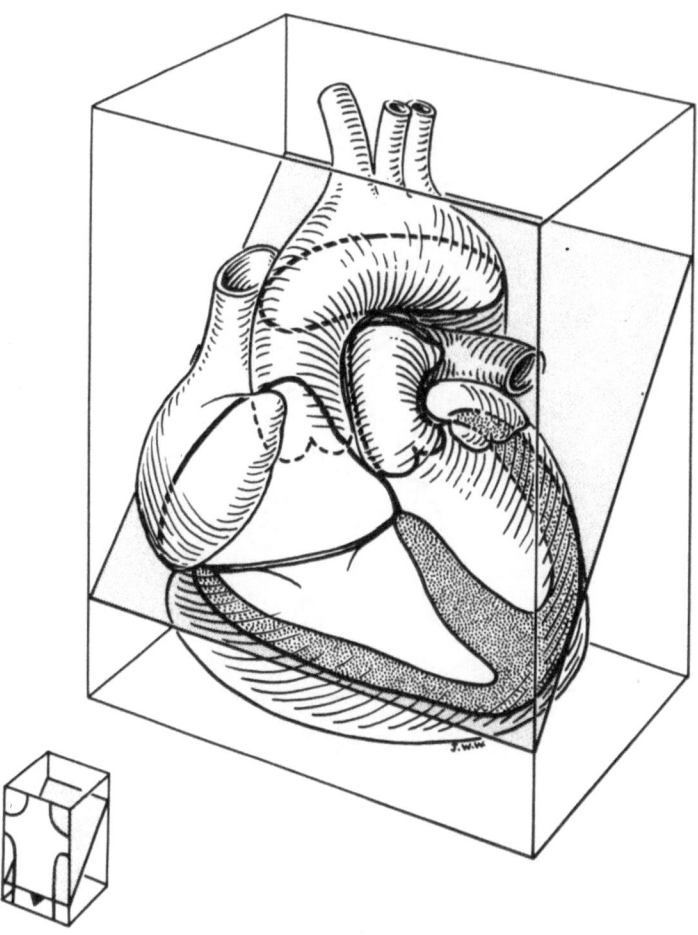

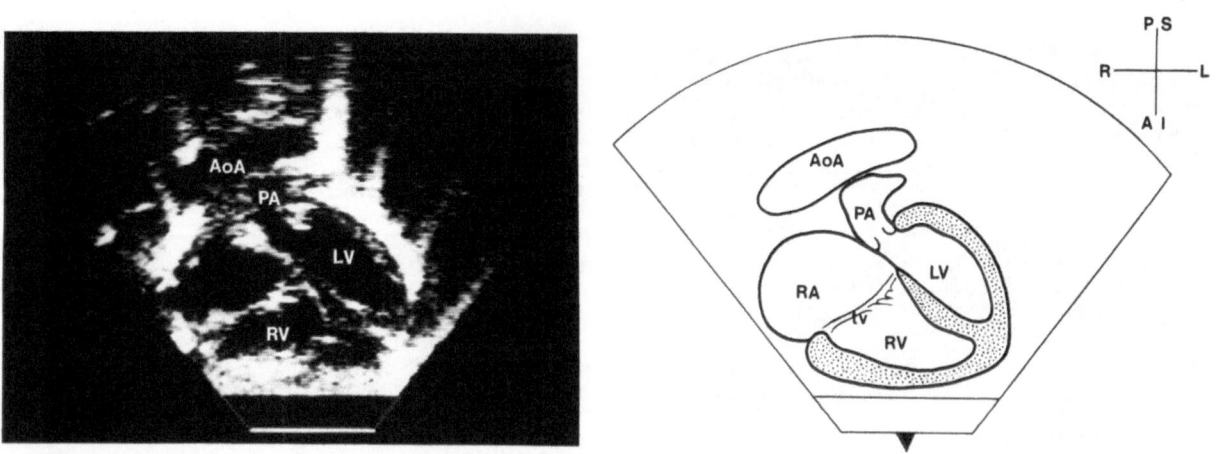

Figure 9.5. Subcostal longitudinal two-dimensional echocardiogram of a patient with transposition of the great arteries. The aortic arch is visualized superior to the pulmonary artery.

AoA = ascending aorta, PA = pulmonary artery, RA = right atrium, tv = tricuspid valve, RV = right ventricle, LV = left ventricle.

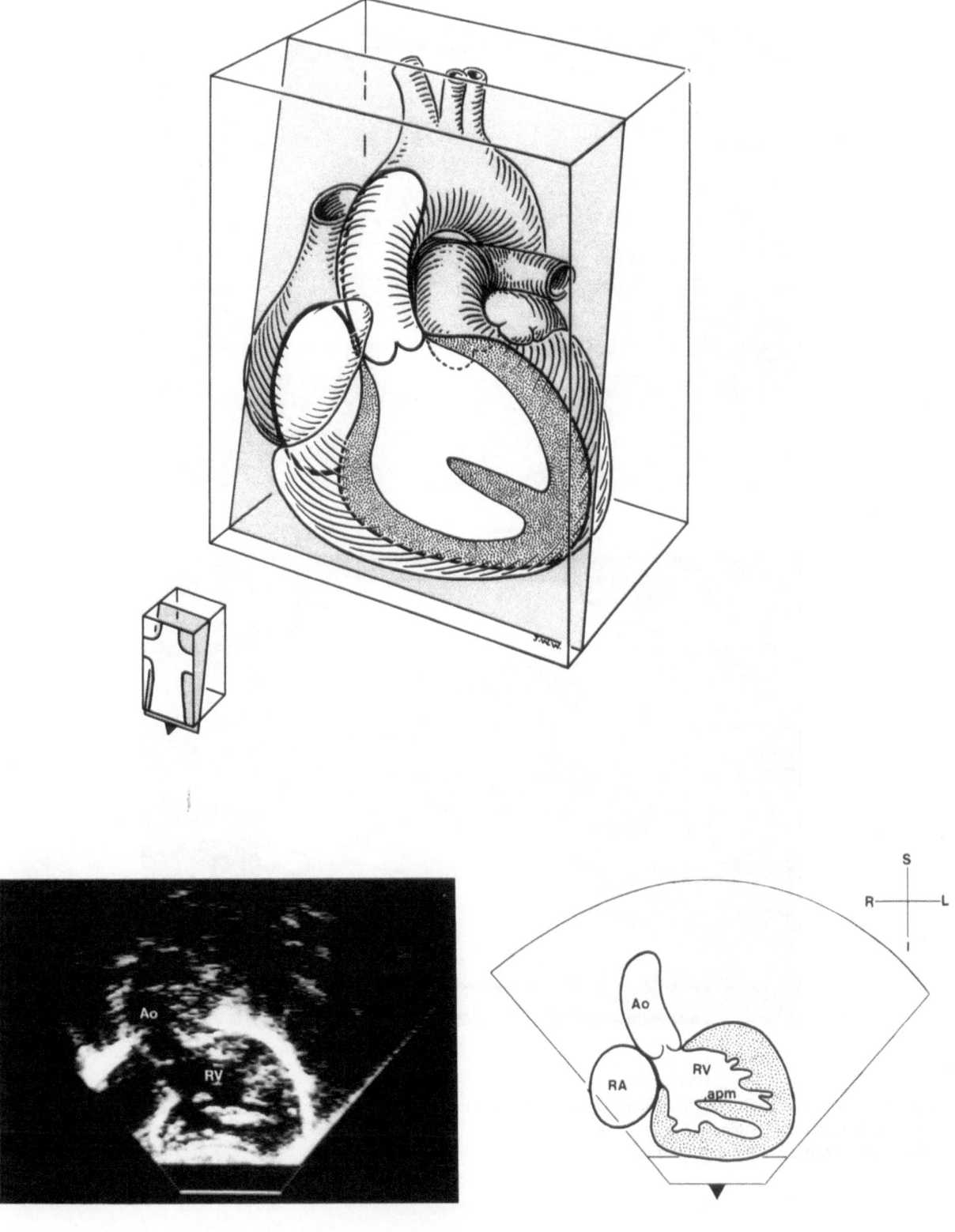

Figure 9.6. Subcostal frontal two-dimensional echocardiogram of the same patient as in Figure 9.5. The ascending aorta originates from the right ventricle.

Ao = *aorta,* RV = *right ventricle,* RA = *right atrium,* apm = *anterior papillary muscle.*

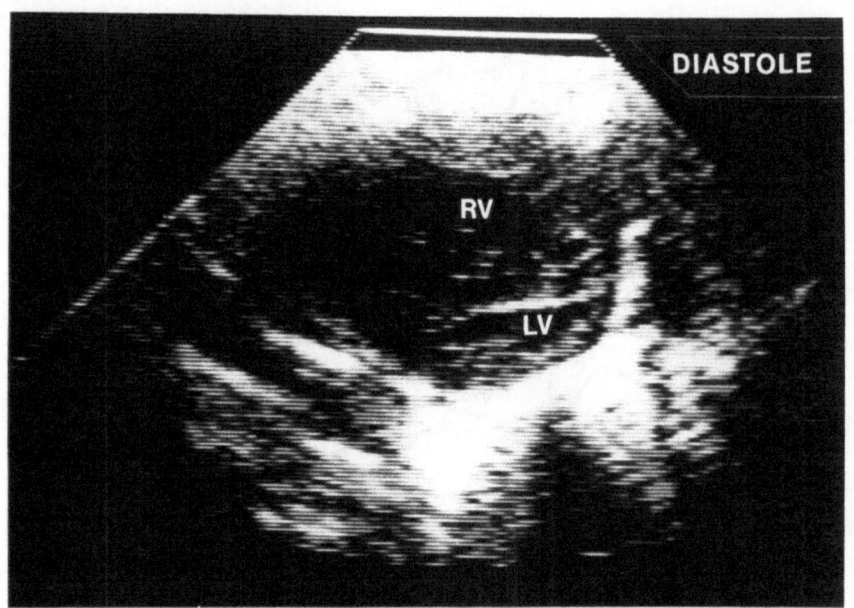

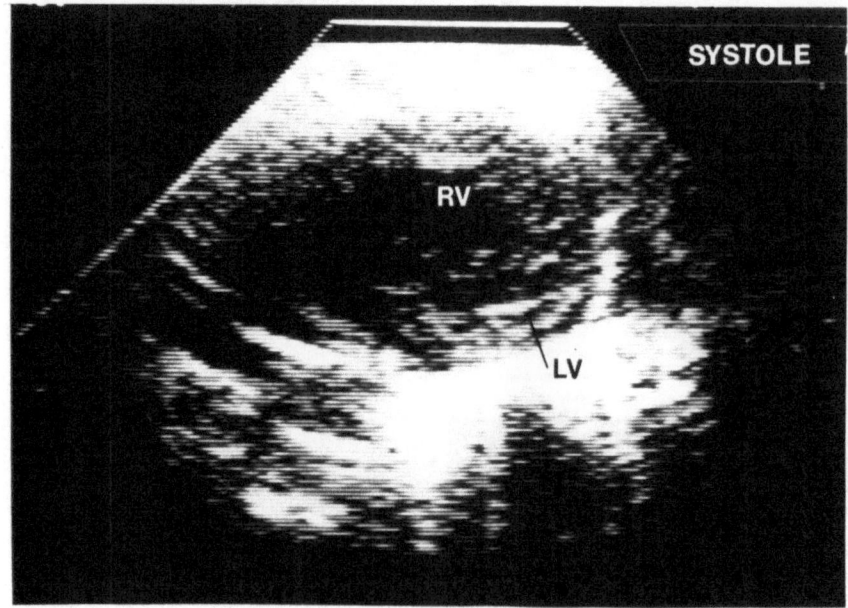

Figure 9.7. Parasternal short axis view of a patient with transposition of the great arteries. The left ventricle is flattened and its cavity is obliterated during systole.

RV = right ventricle, LV = left ventricle.

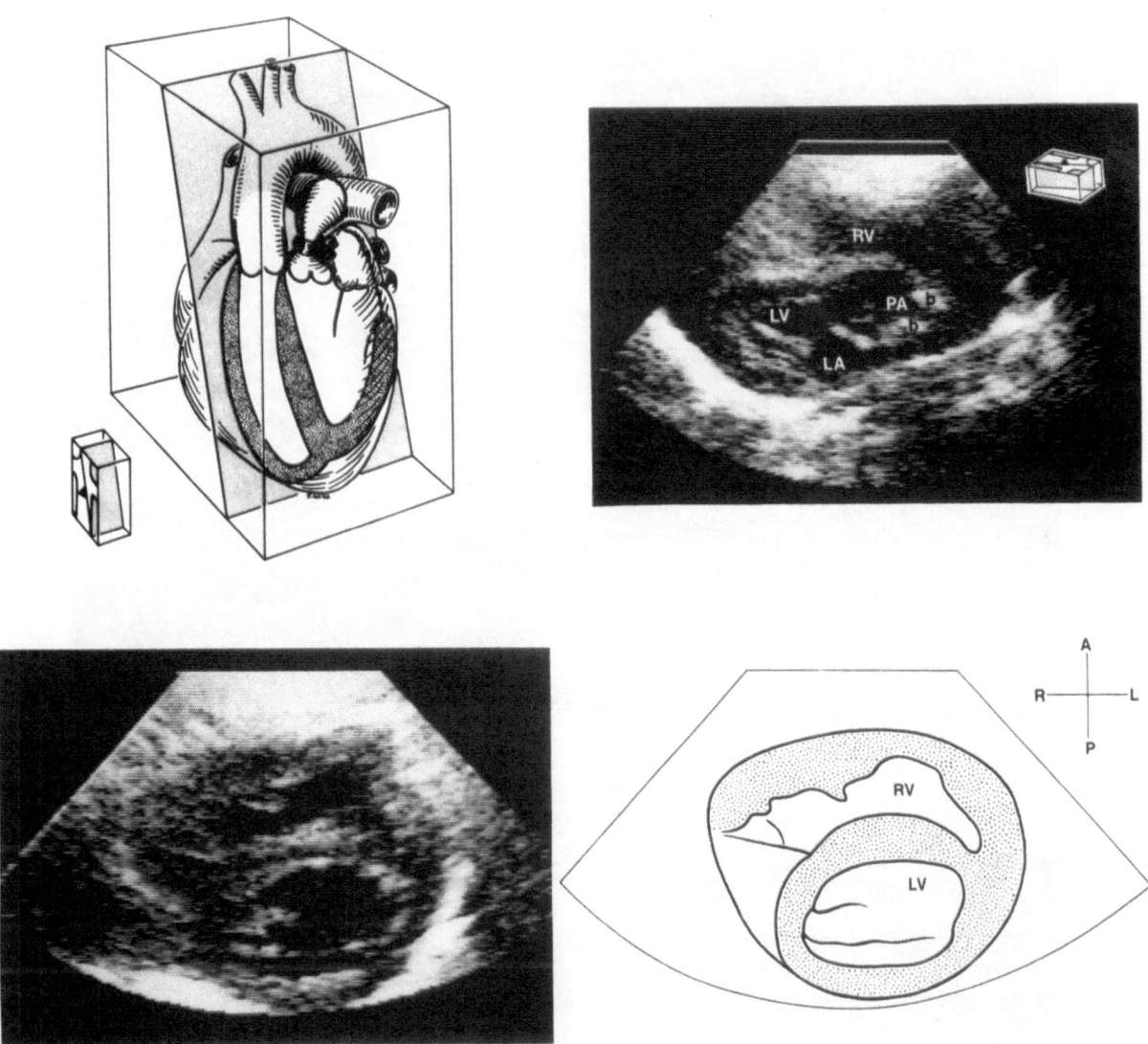

Figure 9.8. Parasternal long axis view (above) and short axis view (below) of a patient with transposition of the great arteries and intact interventricular septum after banding of the pulmonary artery as part of the two-stage anatomical correction. The interventricular septum is convex to the right indicating suprasystemic pressure in the left ventricle.

RV = right ventricle, LV = left ventricle, LA = left atrium, PA = pulmonary artery, b = banding.

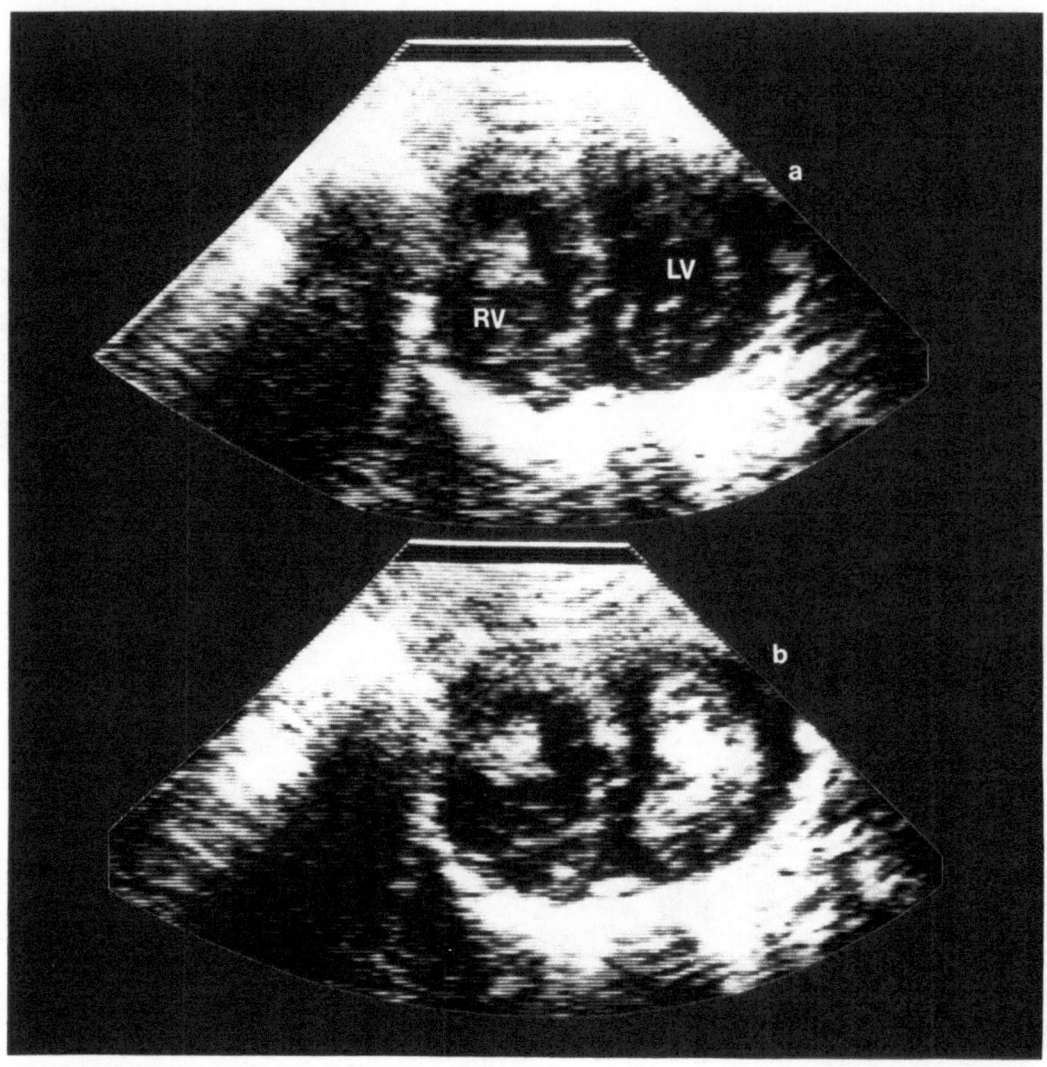

Figure 9.9. Parasternal short axis views of a patient with transposition of the great arteries and intact interventricular septum after preparatory banding of the pulmonary artery and aorto-pulmonary shunt operation. The still frames are taken during end-systole. In panel b the left ventricle is filled with echocontrast which provides an accurate demarcation of the left ventricular endocardial surface. The interventricular septum is slightly convex to the left indicating that the pressure is higher in the right than in the left ventricle. However, the left ventricular dimension and wall thickness are adequately developed.

RV = right ventricle, LV = left ventricle.

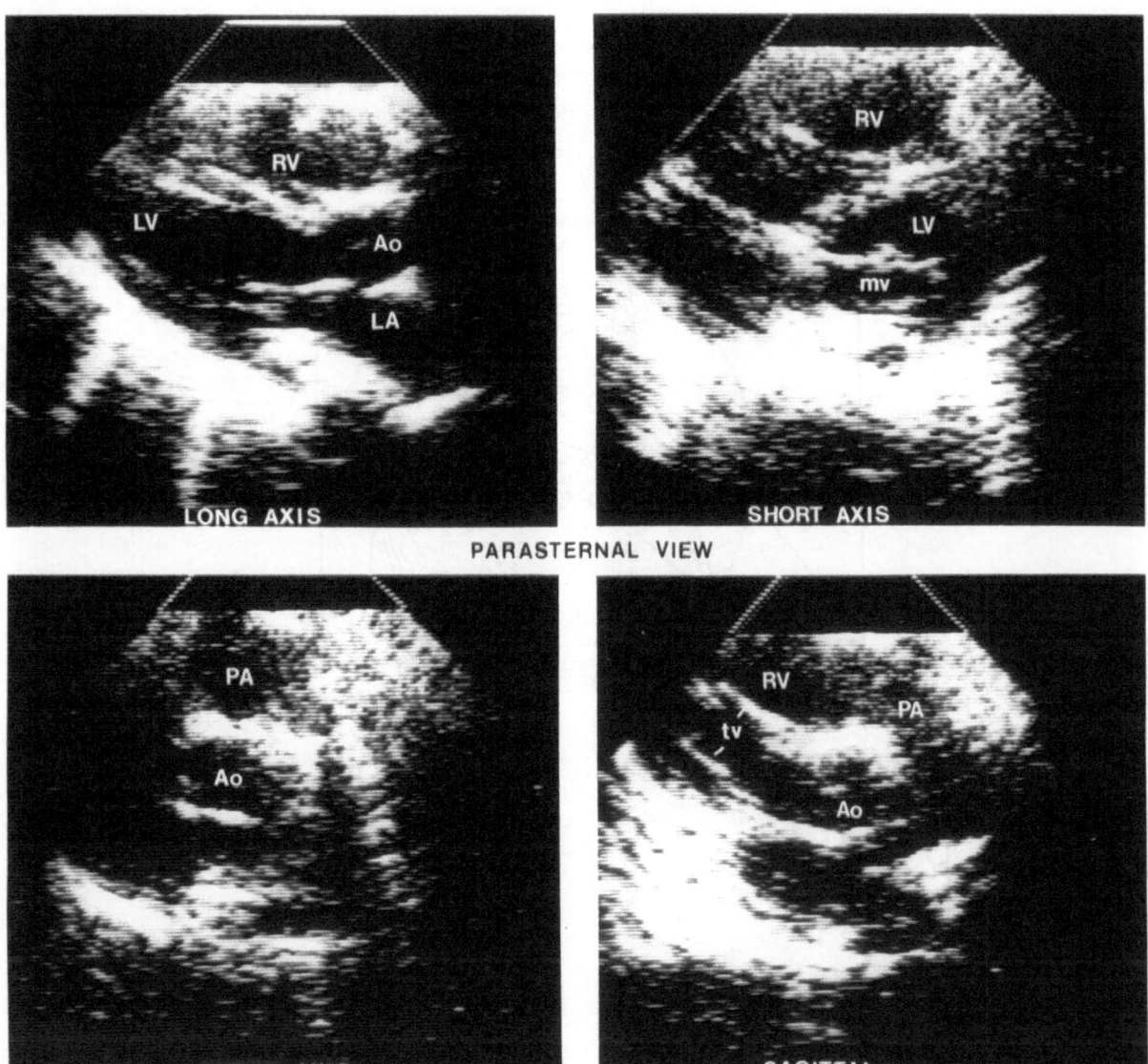

Figure 9.10. Parasternal two-dimensional echocardiograms of a patient with transposition of the great arteries after anatomical correction.

LV = left ventricle, RV = right ventricle, Ao = aorta, LA = left atrium, mv = mitral valve, PA = pulmonary artery, tv = tricuspid valve.

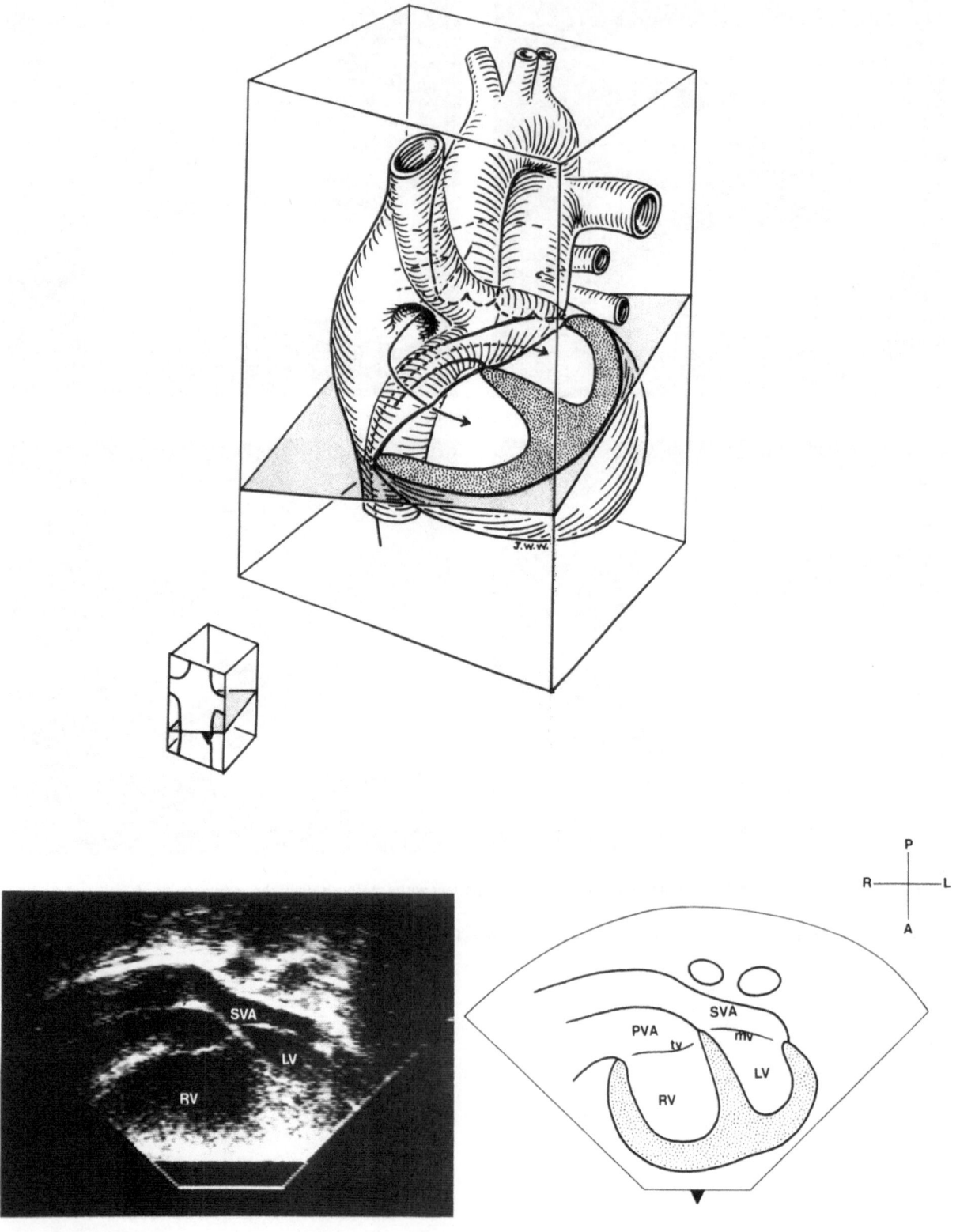

Figure 9.11. Parasternal two-dimensional echocardiogram of a patient with transposition of the great arteries after physiological correction (Mustard-repair). The inferior caval tunnel with its connection to the mitral orifice is visualized.

PVA = pulmonary venous atrium, SVA = systemic venous atrium, tv = tricuspid valve, mv = mitral valve, RV = right ventricle, LV = left ventricle.

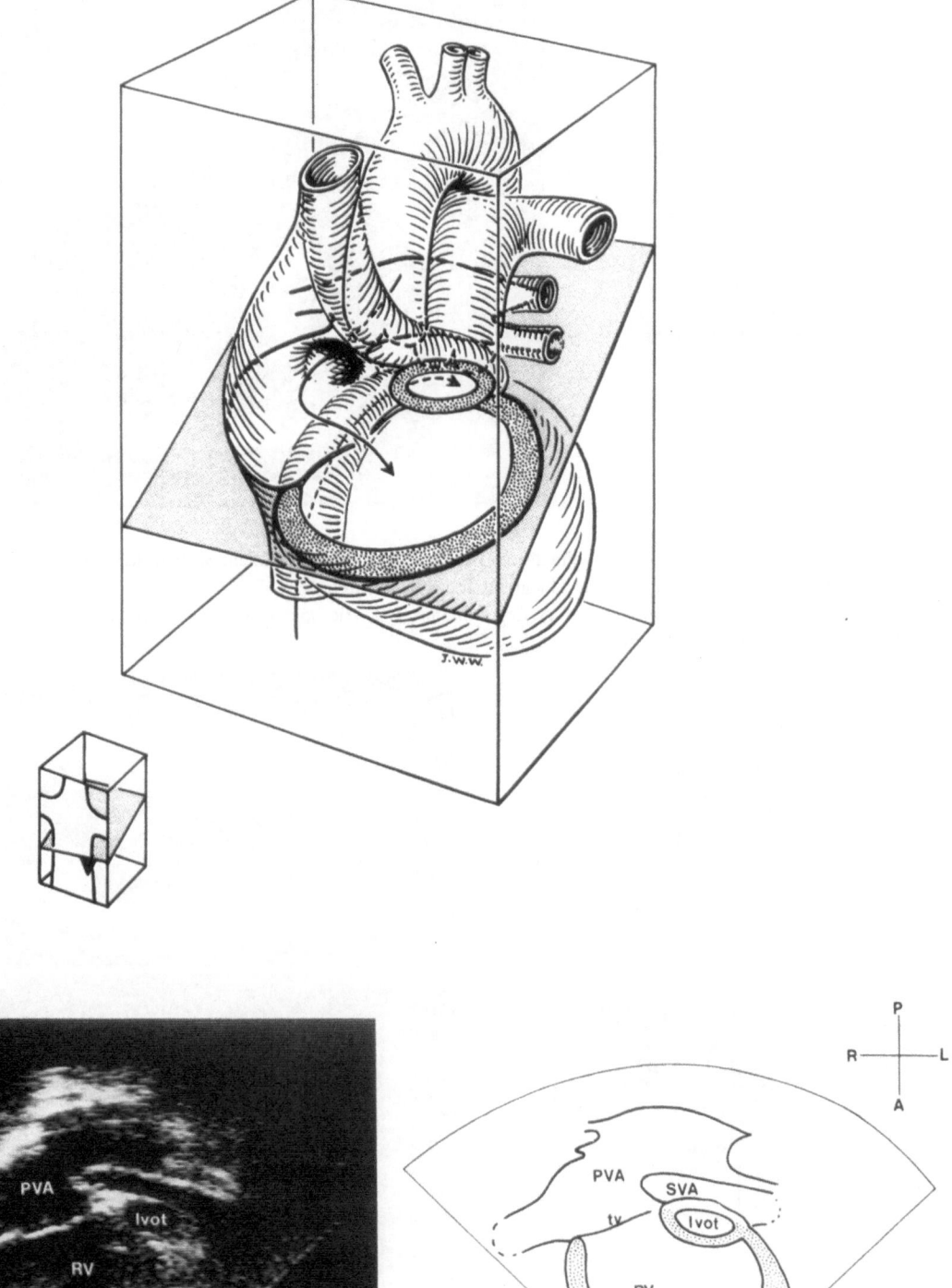

Figure 9.12. Parasternal two-dimensional echocardiogram of the same patient as in Figure 9.11. By tilting the transducer cranially the pulmonary venous atrium is visualized.

PVA = pulmonary venous atrium, SVA = systemic venous atrium, tv = tricuspid valve, lvot = left ventricular outflow tract, RV = right ventricle.

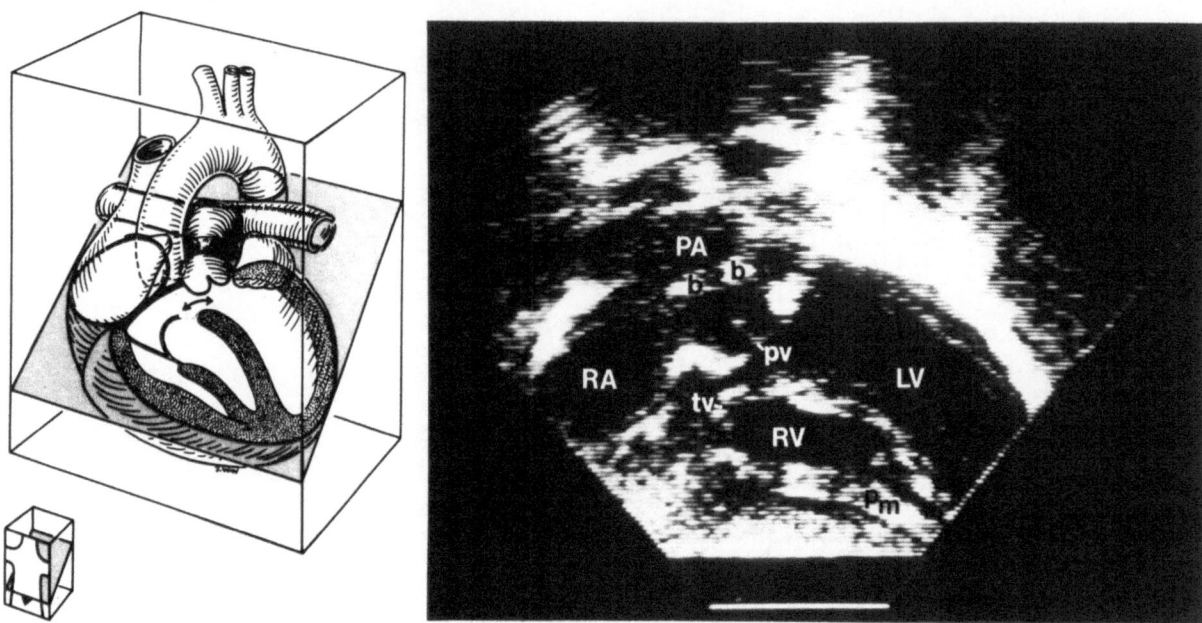

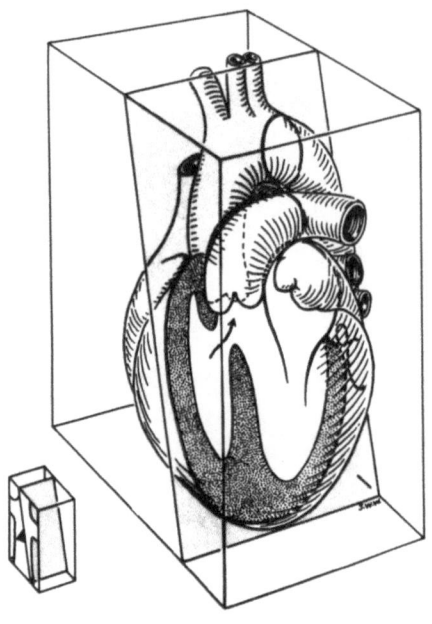

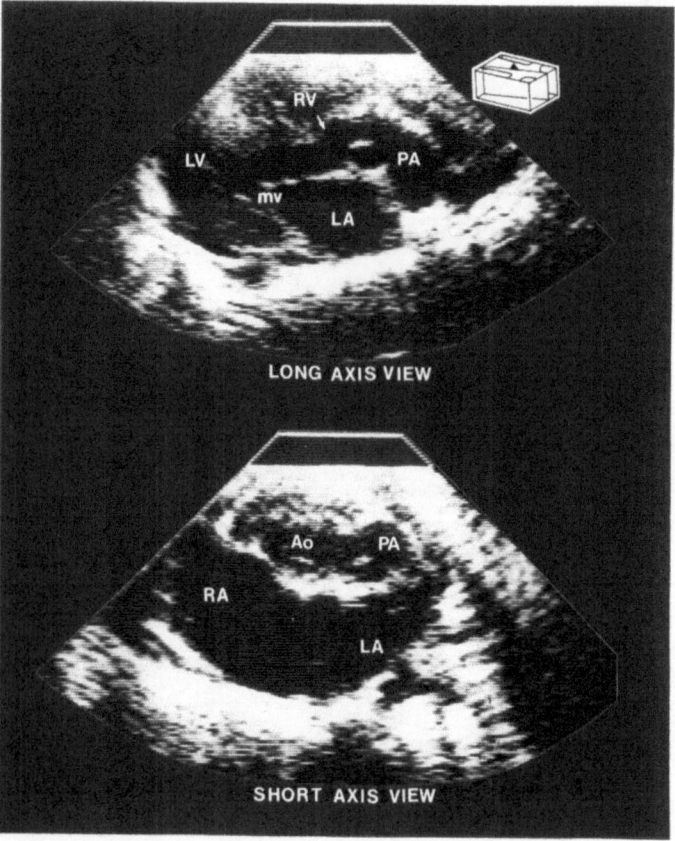

Figure 9.13. Subcostal longitudinal two-dimensional echocardiogram of a patient with transposition of the great arteries and perimembranous ventricular septal defect. The arrow indicates the defect.

RA = right atrium, PA = pulmonary artery, b = banding, tv = tricuspid valve, pv = pulmonary valve, RV = right ventricle, LV = left ventricle, pm = papillary muscle.

Figure 9.14. Parasternal two-dimensional echocardiogram of a patient with transposition of the great arteries and malalignment ventricular septal defect. The arrows indicate the anteriorly located interventricular communication.

LV = left ventricle, RV = right ventricle, LA = left atrium, PA = pulmonary artery, mv = mitral valve, Ao = aorta, RA = right atrium.

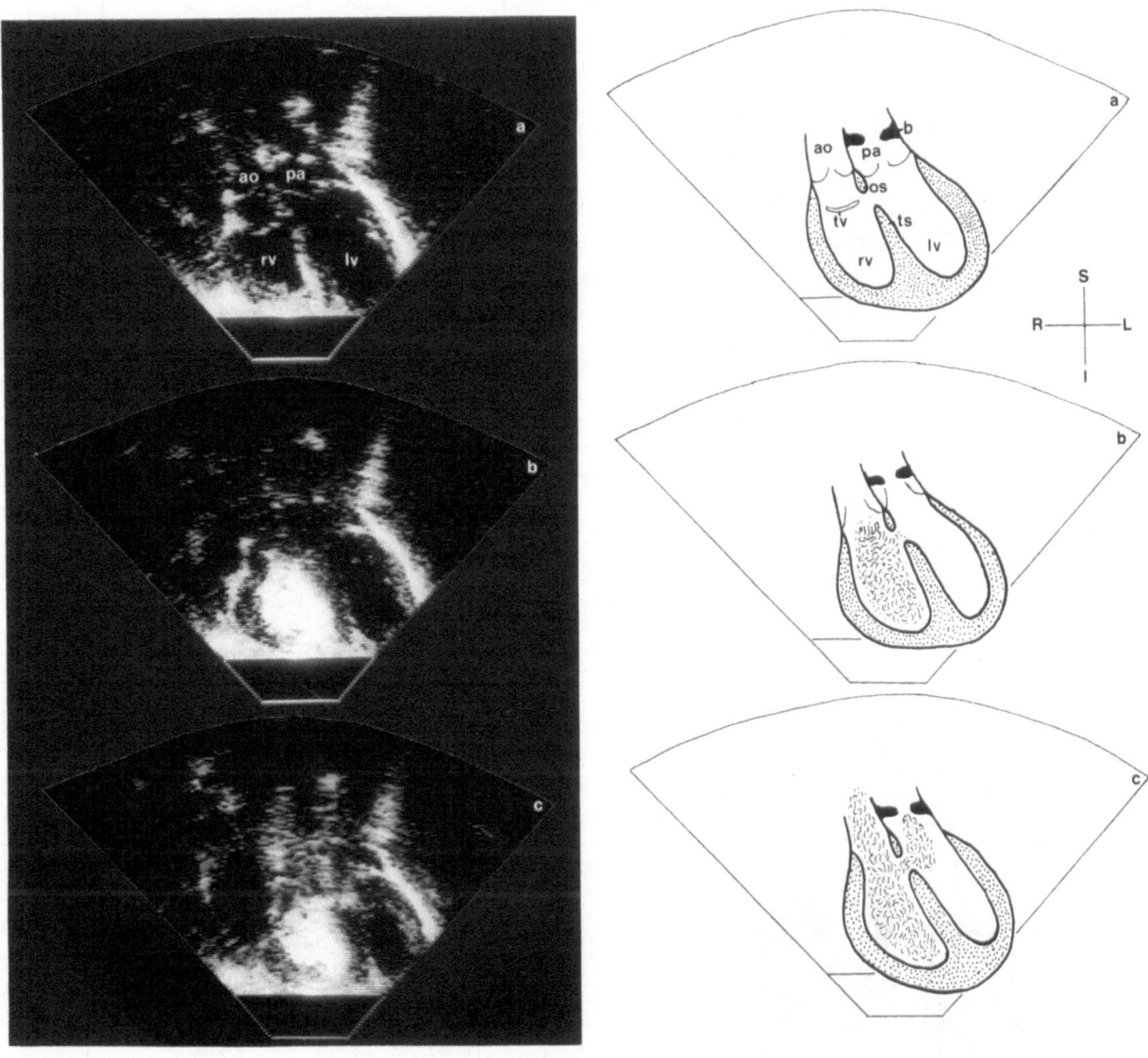

Figure 9.15. Subcostal view of the same patient as in Figure 9.14 before (a) and after (b, c) a venous contrast injection. The pulmonary artery is banded. In panel b the right ventricle is filled with contrast. In panel c the contrast has reached the aorta and has passed the ventricular septal defect towards the left ventricular outflow tract and the proximal part of the pulmonary artery.

ao = aorta, pa = pulmonary artery, b = banding, os = outlet septum, t = trabecular septum, tv = tricuspid valve, rv = right ventricle, lv = left ventricle.

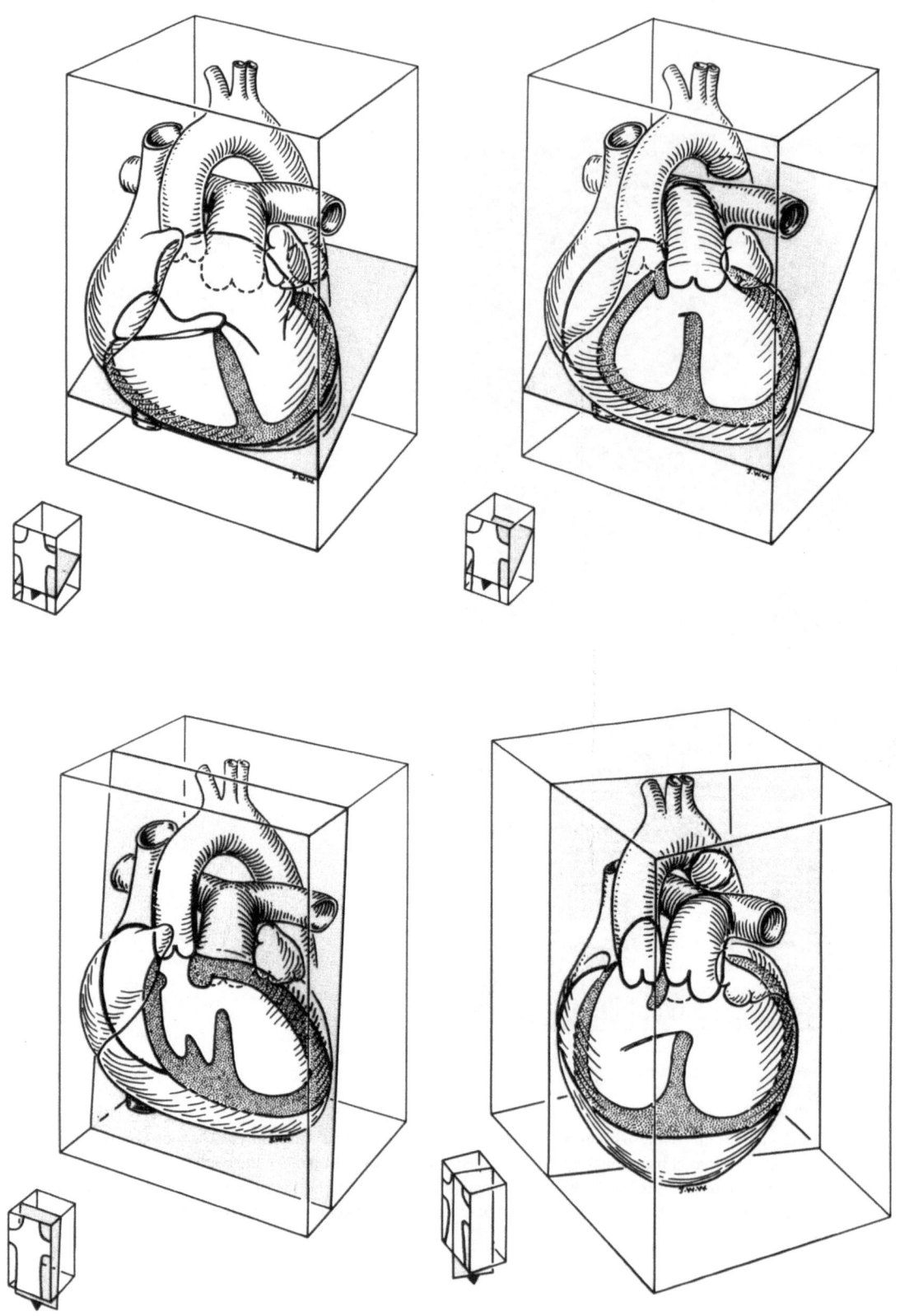

Figure 9.16A. Diagrammatic representation of the two-dimensional echocardiograms of Figure 9.16B.

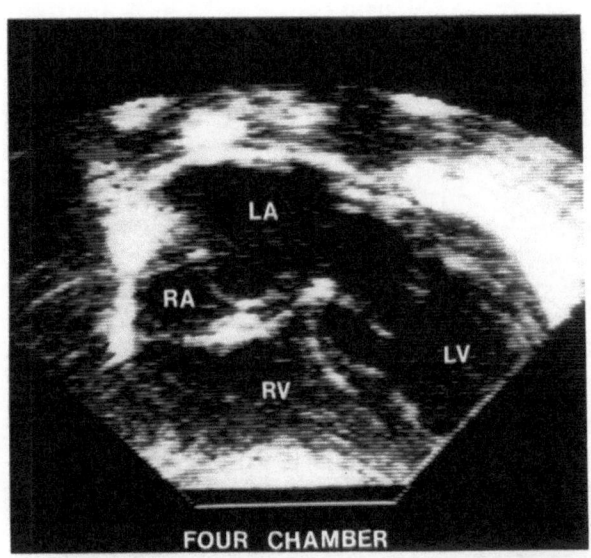

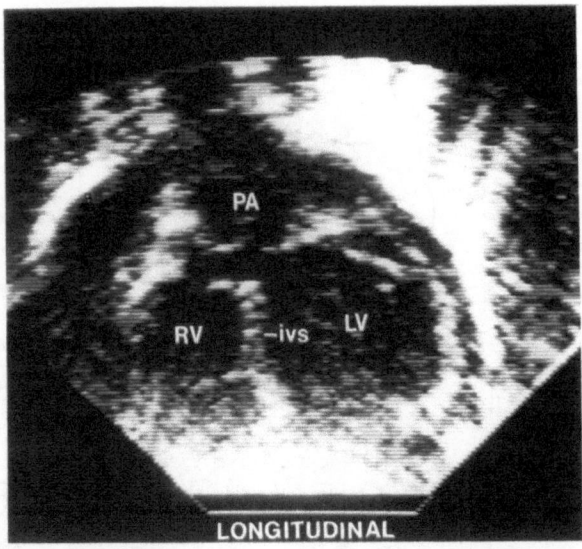

SUBCOSTAL VIEW

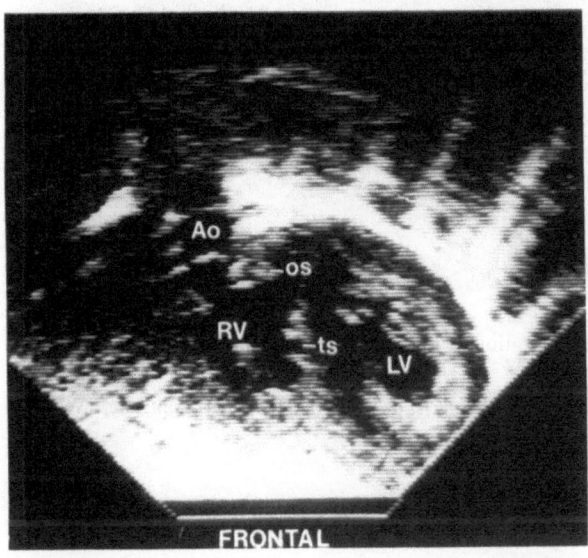

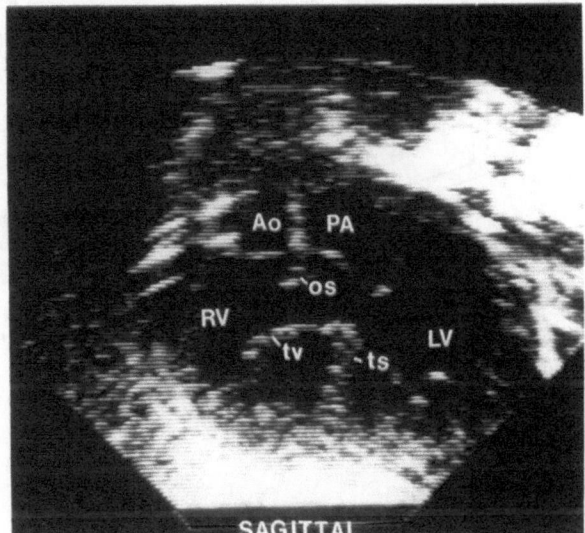

Figure 9.16B. Two-dimensional echocardiograms of a patient with transposition of the great arteries and malalignment ventricular septal defect.

RA = right atrium, LA = left atrium, RV = right ventricle, LV = left ventricle, PA = pulmonary artery, ivs = interventricular septum, Ao = aorta, os = outlet septum, ts = trabecular septum, tv = tricuspid valve.

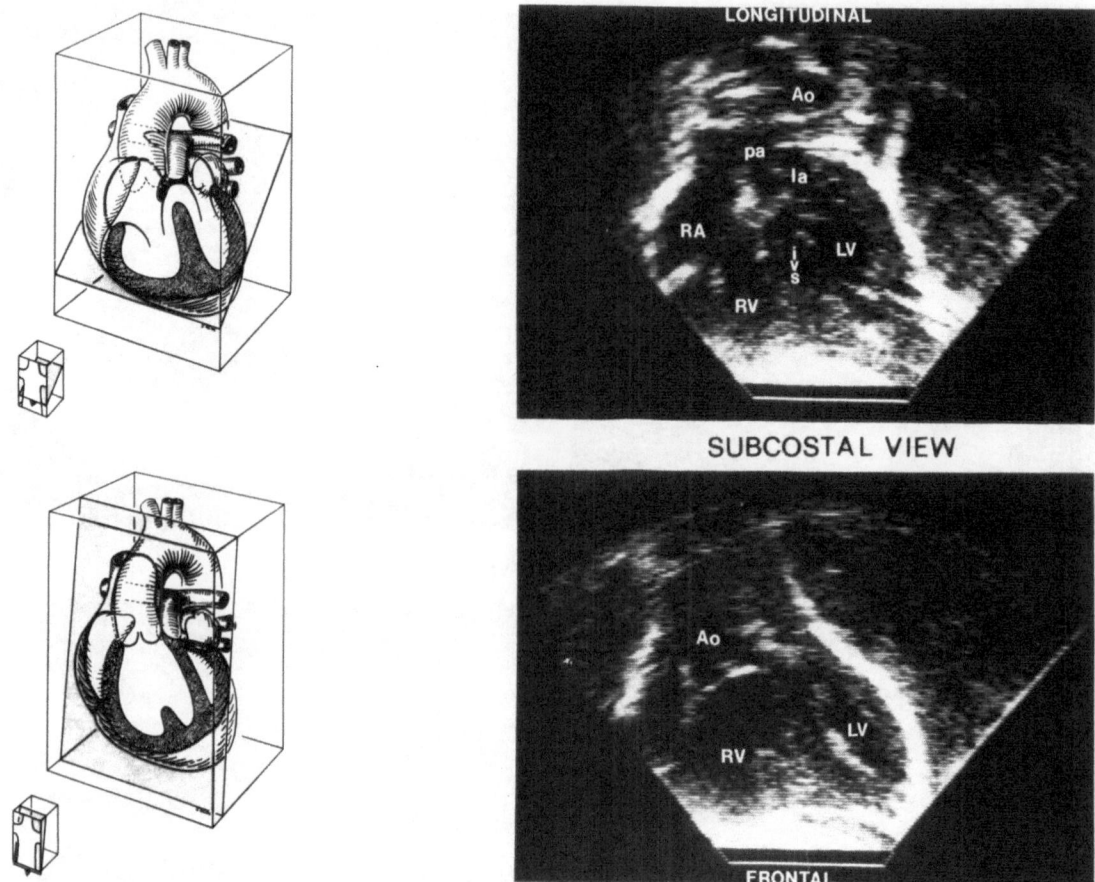

Figure 9.17. Two-dimensional echocardiograms of a patient with transposition of the great arteries, ventricular septal defect and pulmonary stenosis.

Ao = aorta, pa = pulmonary artery, la = left atrium, RA = right atrium, RV = right ventricle, LV = left ventricle, IVS = interventricular septum.

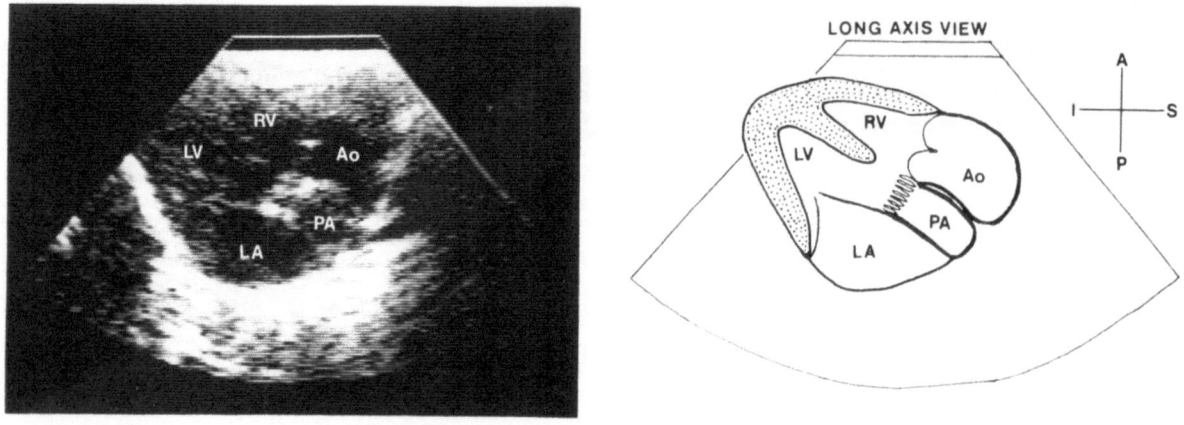

Figure 9.18. Two-dimensional echocardiogram of the same patient as in Figure 9.17.

LV = left ventricle, RV = right ventricle, Ao = aorta, PA = pulmonary artery, LA = left atrium.

10. AORTIC STENOSIS

Severe aortic valvular stenosis, like severe pulmonary valvular stenosis is particularly amenable to non-invasive diagnosis. A rough systolic ejection murmur of low frequency radiating along the course of the aorta towards the carotid arteries with maximal intensity at the second right intercostal space will always be present unless the patient is in severe congestive heart failure. Immediately preceding the cardiac murmur an ejection click is normally heard. The electrocardiogram provides valuable information when the left ventricular hypertrophy, based on voltage criteria, is associated with ST-T abnormalities.

Two-dimensional echocardiography easily visualizes the centrally located aortic valve and abnormalities are readily detected. The thickening of the aortic valve is particularly evident during diastole. The diastolic closure line of a normal aortic valve appears in the parasternal long axis view as a single and thin line in the centre of the aorta parallel to the aortic walls. In aortic stenosis the diastole frequently reveals a thick closure line perpendicular to the walls of the aorta (Figure 10.1). The severity of the stenosis is best appreciated during systole when the dome-shape of the valve with its superior opening is visualized. The diameter of this opening approximates the severity of the stenosis (1). Figure 10.2 displays the echocardiograms of a patient with critical aortic valvular stenosis before and after commissurotomy. The preoperative echocardiogram shows the extreme limitation of the leaflet separation during systole. The dilatation of the left ventricular cavity is more striking than the thickness of the wall of the left ventricle. This corresponded with the presence of overt heart failure in this patient. Postoperatively, the valve leaflets come much further apart. The left ventricular cavity is much smaller and the wall thickness is increased. Figure 10.3 shows the echocardiogram of another patient with aortic stenosis but without cardiac failure. The considerably increased left ventricular wall thickness suggests a critical stenosis. The long axis still frame does not adequately show the aortic valve leaflets. The diastolic closure line is vaguely visible and is perpendicular to the walls of the aorta. The ascending aorta shows a widening of the lumen superior to the valve due to poststenotic dilatation. In the short axis the 'Mercedes' sign reveals the tricuspid nature of this aortic valve (Figure 10.4).

A frequently occurring anomaly of the aortic apparatus is bicuspid aortic valve. This may be associated with stenosis of the valve but in the majority of the cases it has hardly any or no haemodynamic consequences. A bicuspid aortic valve, visualized in the long axis and short axis views, is displayed in Figure 10.5. The diastolic closure line is seen in the aortic root, parallel to the walls of the aorta. Compared with the normal it is displaced anteriorly, i.e. nearer the anterior wall of the aorta, because the anterior cusp is smaller than the posterior one. The short axis view shows how the closure line bridges in a straight line the entire breadth of the aortic circle, connecting the right and left sides (2). This observation is indicative of a bicuspid aortic valve.

A discrete subvalvular membranous or fibromuscular aortic stenosis also produces an ejection murmur but its maximal intensity is, unlike that of valvular aortic stenosis, at the left lower sternal border and there is no ejection click. The membrane of fibromuscular ridge is usually best visualized in the parasternal long axis view (3) (Figure 10.6). Another echocardiographic approach is to visualize the lesion in the apical long axis view as reported by DiSessa et al (4). Two-dimensional echocardiography is also valuable for the detection of the supra-valvular aortic stenosis (5).

116

References

1. Weyman AE, Feigenbaum H, Hurwitz RA, Girod DA, Dillon JC: Cross-sectional echocardiographic assessment of the severity of aortic stenosis in children. Circulation 55:773 – 778, 1977.
2. Bansal RS, Tajik AJ, Seward JB, Offord KP: Feasibility of detailed two-dimensional echocardiographic examination in adults. Prospective study of 200 patients. Mayo Clin Proc 55:291 – 308, 1980.
3. Wilcox WD, Seward JB, Hagler DJ, Mair DD, Tajik AJ: Discrete subaortic stenosis, two-dimensional echocar-diographic features with angiographic and surgical correlation. Mayo Clin Proc 55:425 – 433, 1980.
4. DiSessa TG, Hagan AD, Isabel-Jones JB, Ti CC, Mercier JC, Friedman WF: Two-dimensional echocardiographic evaluation of discrete subaortic stenosis from the apical long axis view. Am Heart J 101:774 – 782, 1981.
5. Weyman AE, Caldwell RL, Hurwitz RA, Girod DA, Dillon JC, Feigenbaum H, Green D: Cross-sectional echocardiographic characterization of aortic obstruction, supravalvular aortic stenosis and aortic hypoplasia. Circulation 57:491 – 497, 1977.

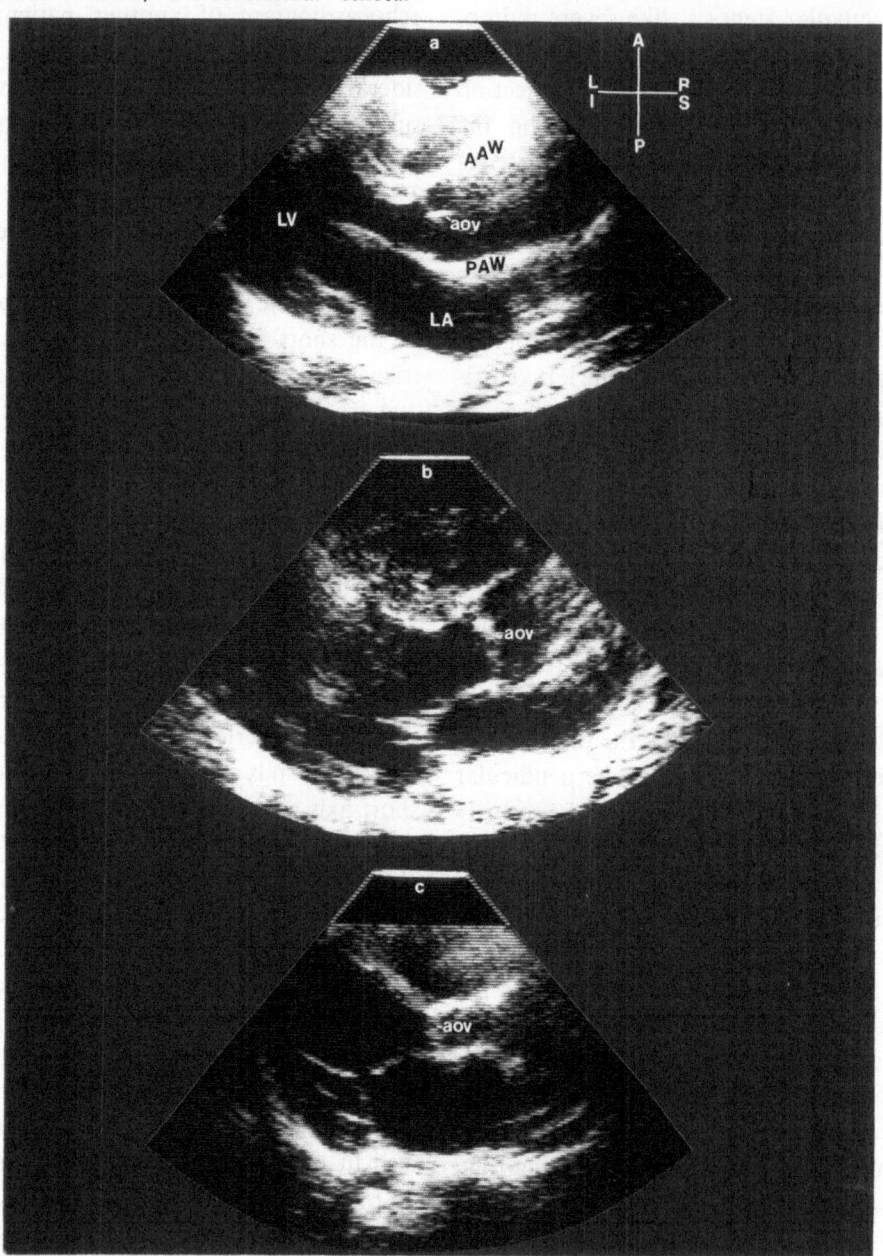

Figure 10.1. Parasternal long axis two-dimensional echocardiograms. Diastolic still frames are shown. The closure line of the non-stenotic aortic valve in a patient with idiopatic aortic dilatation discloses a normal course parallel to the aortic walls (a). The next echocardiogram (b) shows the closure line of a stenotic aortic valve in an older boy. It lies perpendicular to the aortic walls. A similar echocardiogram is displayed of an infant (c).

AAW = anterior aortic wall, PAW = posterior aortic wall, aov = aortic valve, LV = left ventricle, LA = left atrium.

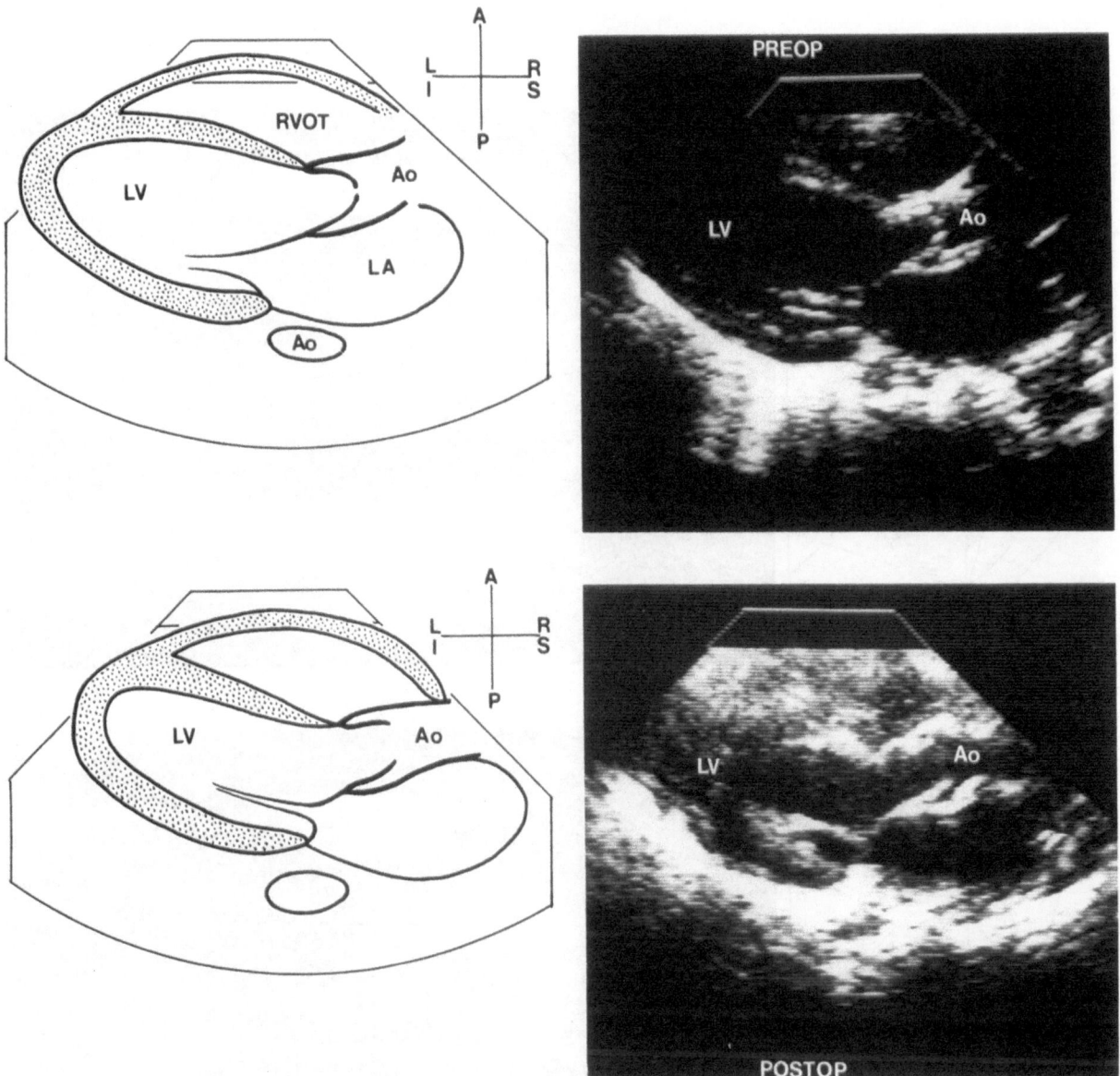

Figure 10.2. Parasternal long axis two-dimensional echocardiograms of a patient with severe valvular aortic stenosis before and after operation.

RVOT = right ventricular outflow tract, LV = left ventricle, Ao = aorta, LA = left atrium.

118

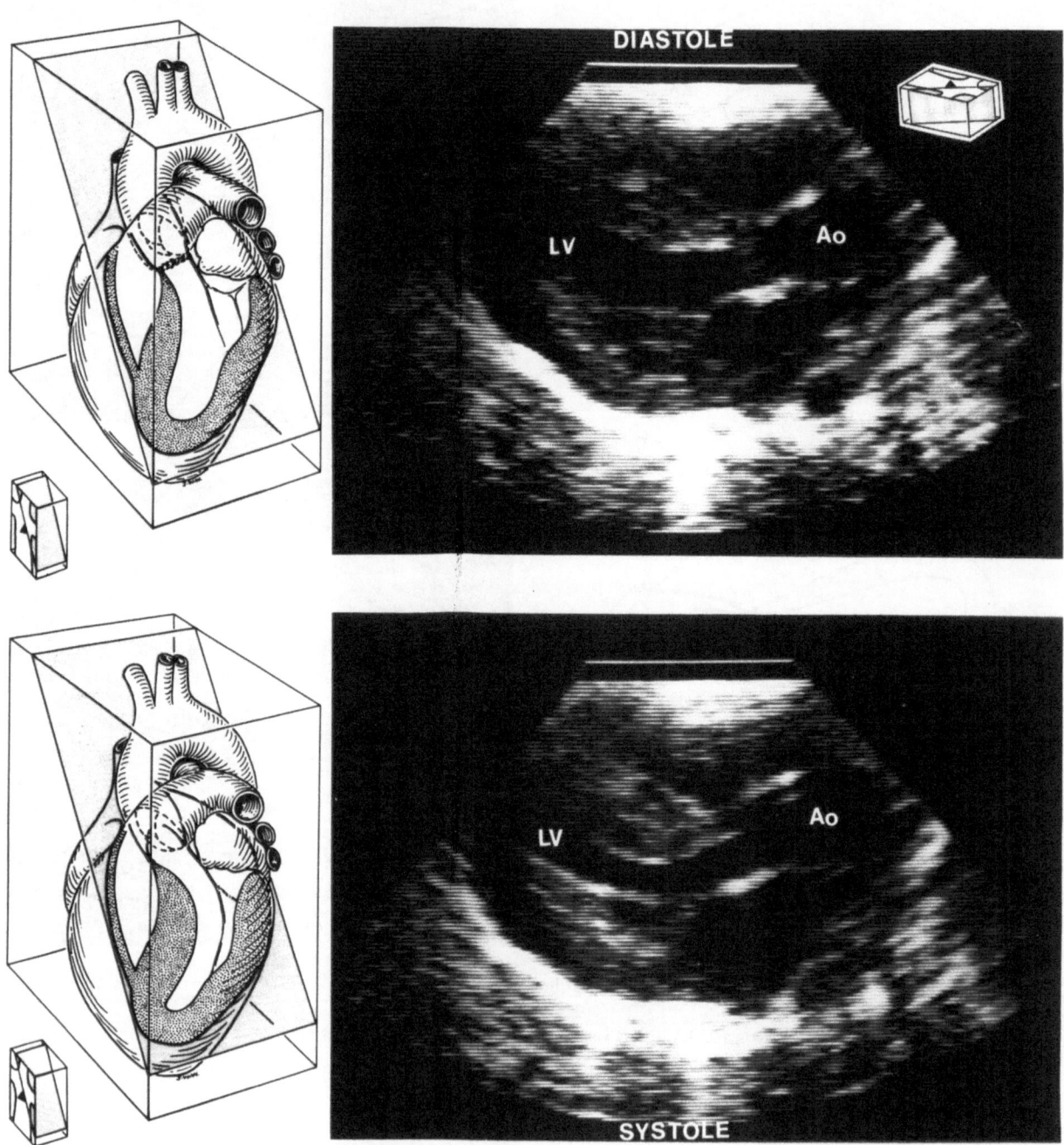

Figure 10.3. Parasternal long axis two-dimensional echocardiogram of a patient with severe valvular aortic stenosis.
LV = left ventricle, Ao = aorta.

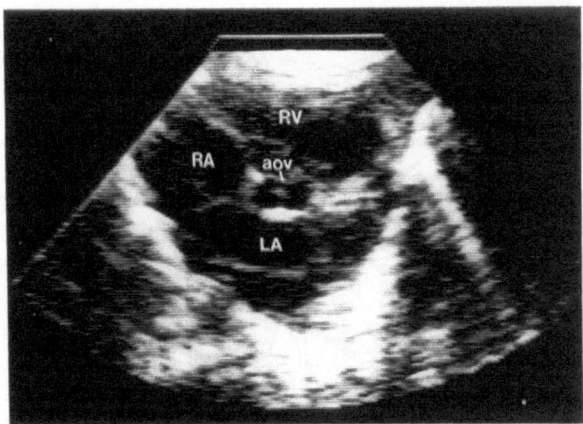

Figure 10.4. Parasternal short axis two-dimensional echocardiogram of the same patient as in Figure 10.3.
RV = right ventricle, RA = right atrium, LA = left atrium, aov = aortic valve.

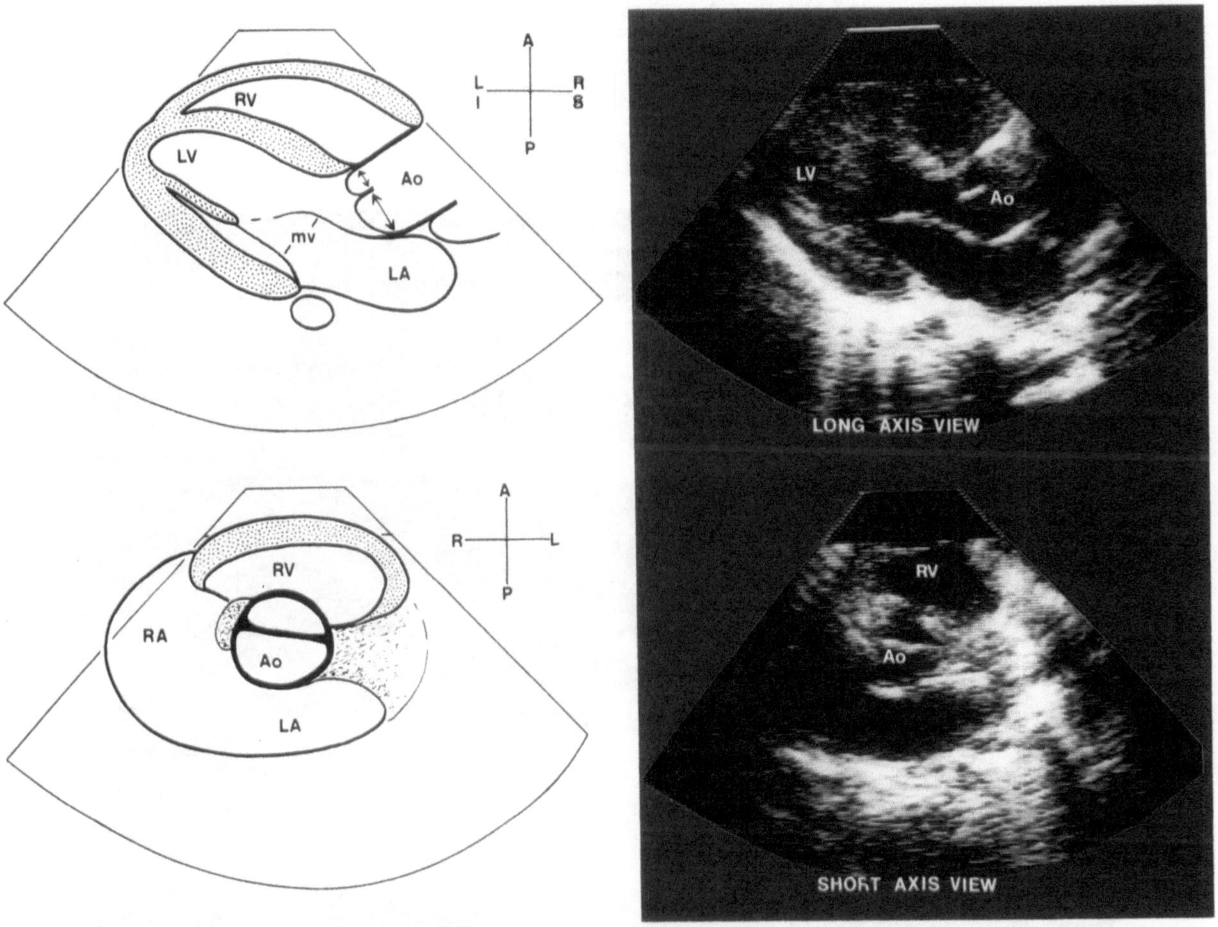

Figure 10.5. Parasternal two-dimensional echocardiogram of a patient with a bicuspid aortic valve.
RV = right ventricle, LV = left ventricle, Ao = aorta, LA = left atrium, RA = right atrium, mv = mitral valve.

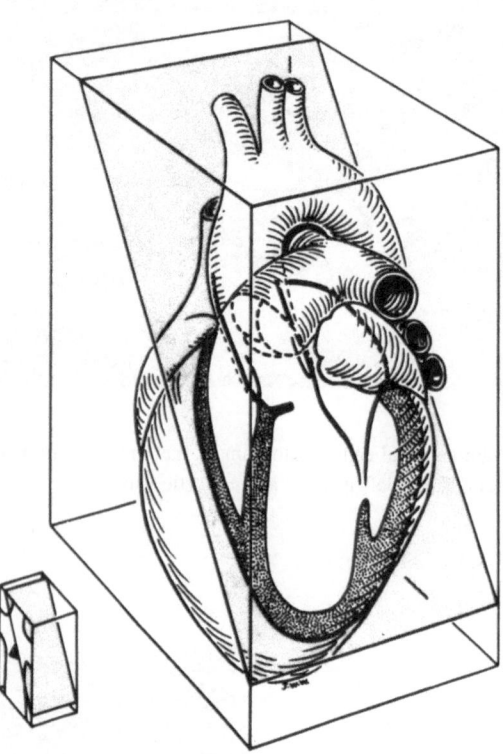

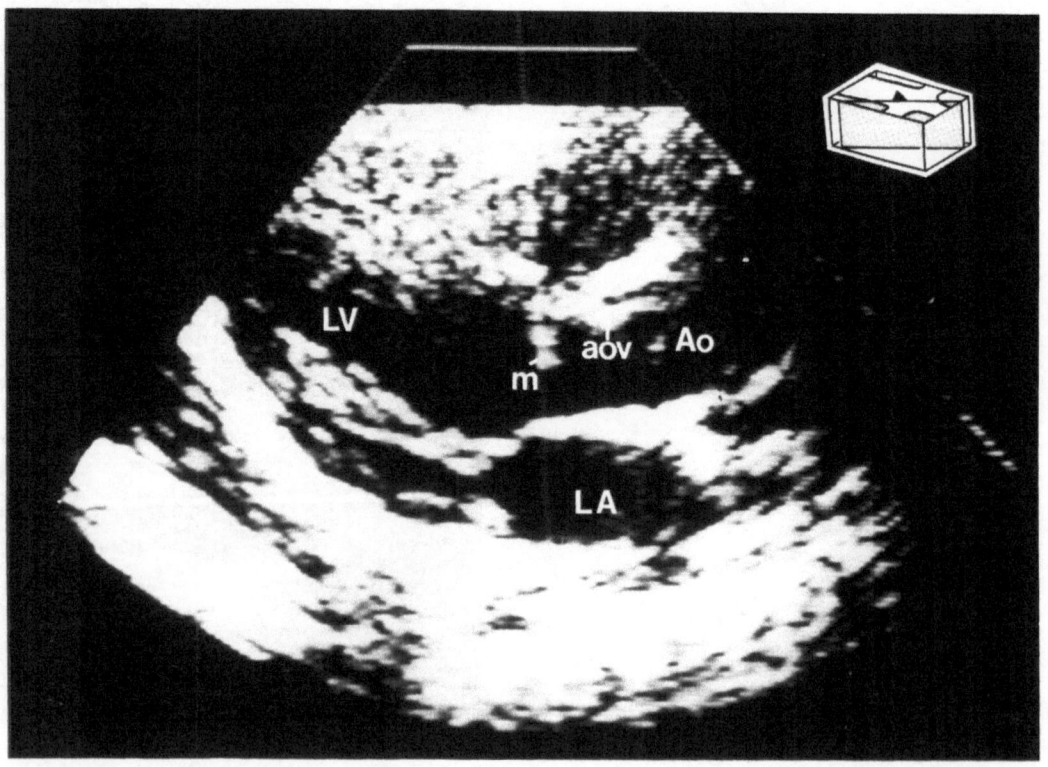

Figure 10.6. Parasternal long axis two-dimensional echocardiogram of a patient with discrete subaortic stenosis.
LV = left ventricle, LA = left atrium, Ao = aorta, aov = aortic valve, m = membrane or fibromuscular ridge.

11. HYPOPLASTIC LEFT HEART

In hypoplastic left heart syndrome the left ventricle is usually extremely underdeveloped. The mitral valve is rudimentary structure and the aortic orifice is atretic. The pulmonary venous blood essentially flows from the left atrium to the right atrium. As the systemic blood flow depends entirely on patency of the ductus arteriosus, closure of the ductus soon after birth threathens life. On presentation the infant is extremely pale and cyanotic. Arterial pulsations are faint or absent. The clinical picture simulates shock associated with septicaemia or severe acidosis. The electrocardiogram shows little or no left ventricular activity and the chest X-ray reveals cardiomegaly with increased pulmonary vascular markings or with pulmonary venous congestion. These findings suggest hypoplastic left heart syndrome.

The diagnosis can be confirmed by two-dimensional echocardiography (1). The cardiomegaly is due to dilatation of the right atrium and the right ventricle. The atrial septum may bulge to the right indicating a restrictive foramen ovale. The hypoplastic left ventricle should be looked for posteriorly, superior to the right ventricle. Figure 11.1 and 11.2 display the four chamber view and the long axis view of a hypoplastic left heart whereby the latter view visualizes a small ascending aorta. Real-time imaging showed that the minute left ventricle did not contract itself but moved passively with the right ventricle. There was no continuity between the cavity of left ventricle and the cavity of the ascending aorta indicating aortic atresia. Communication between the left atrium and the left ventricle was seen in the four chamber view. Figure 11.3 and 11.4 show similar cross-sections of another example of hypoplastic left heart with a markedly thickened left ventricular wall. Real-time imaging did not reveal left ventricular contractions *in this case either. A discontinuity of the left ven-*tricular wall was seen on the atrial side. At this site the long axis view revealed the rudiment of the mitral valve. Apparently, there was extreme underdevelopment of the ascending aorta as it could not be traced in the long axis view. Sometimes the ascending aorta can be seen in the short axis view, at the level of the great arteries, even when significantly underdeveloped (Figure 11.5).

In hypoplastic left heart the left ventricular cavity does not have the normal elliptical but a spherical shape (2). This phenomenon can clearly be observed in the presented cases.

Less severe forms of hypoplastic left heart may also occur. They must be distinguished from other defects associated with underdeveloped left ventricles e.g. coarctation of the aorta and cor triatriatum. Therefore, the shape, size and function of the left ventricle and the presence and motion of the mitral and aortic valves should be carefully observed. Severe acidosis in the presence of such lesions may negatively influence cardiac function and as such erroneously suggest hypoplastic left heart. Hence, if in doubt the investigation should be repeated after correction of the acidosis.

Latson and associates (2) measured the cross-sectional area of the left ventricle from the long axis view. An area of 1.6 cm² or less in a newborn infant weighing approximately 3 kg indicates hypoplasia of the left ventricle not compatible with life.

The examiner should be aware of the occurrence of rare defects associated with the hypoplastic left heart syndrome. These are mitral atresia with moderately developed aorta and left ventricle and aortic atresia with reasonably well developed left ventricle and mitral valve. These cases are always associated with a ventricular septal defect. Although literature and personal information on these cases are missing, there are no reasons to

122

suspect difficulties with the two-dimensional echocardiographic recognition of these cases.

References

1. Lange LW, Sahn DJ, Allen HD, Ovitt TW, Goldber SJ: Cross-sectional echocardiography in hypoplastic left ventricle: echocardiographic-angiographic- anatomic correlations. Ped Cardiol 1:287–299, 1980.
2. Latson LA, Cheatham JP, Gutgesell HP: Relation of the echocardiographic estimate of left ventricular size to mortality in infants with severe left ventricular outflow obstruction. Am J Card 48:887–891, 1981.

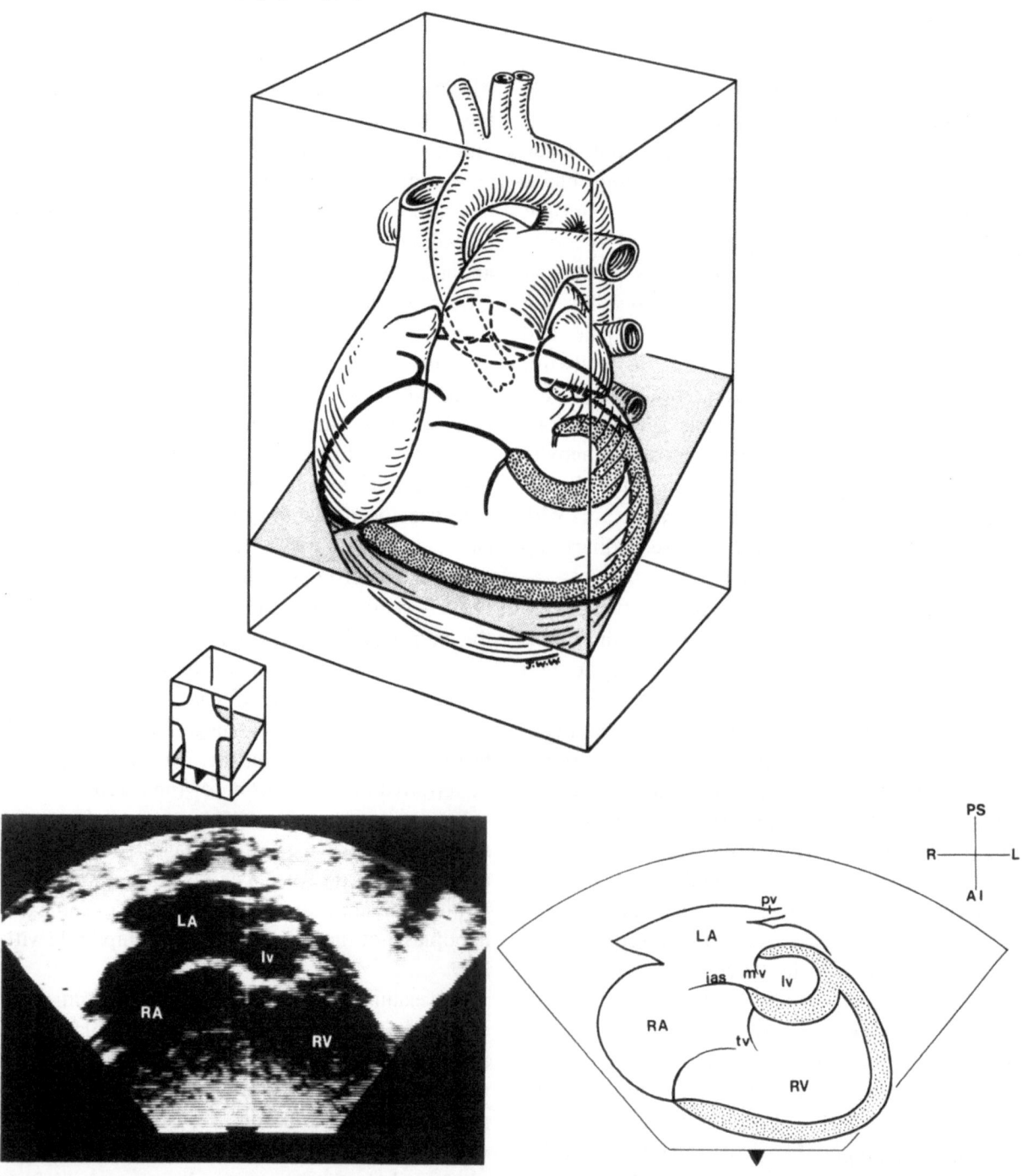

Figure 11.1. Subcostal four chamber two-dimensional echocardiogram of an infant with hypoplastic left heart syndrome.
LA = left atrium, lv = left ventricle, RA = right atrium, RV = right ventricle, pv = pulmonary vein, ias = interatrial septum, mv = mitral valve, tv = tricuspid valve.

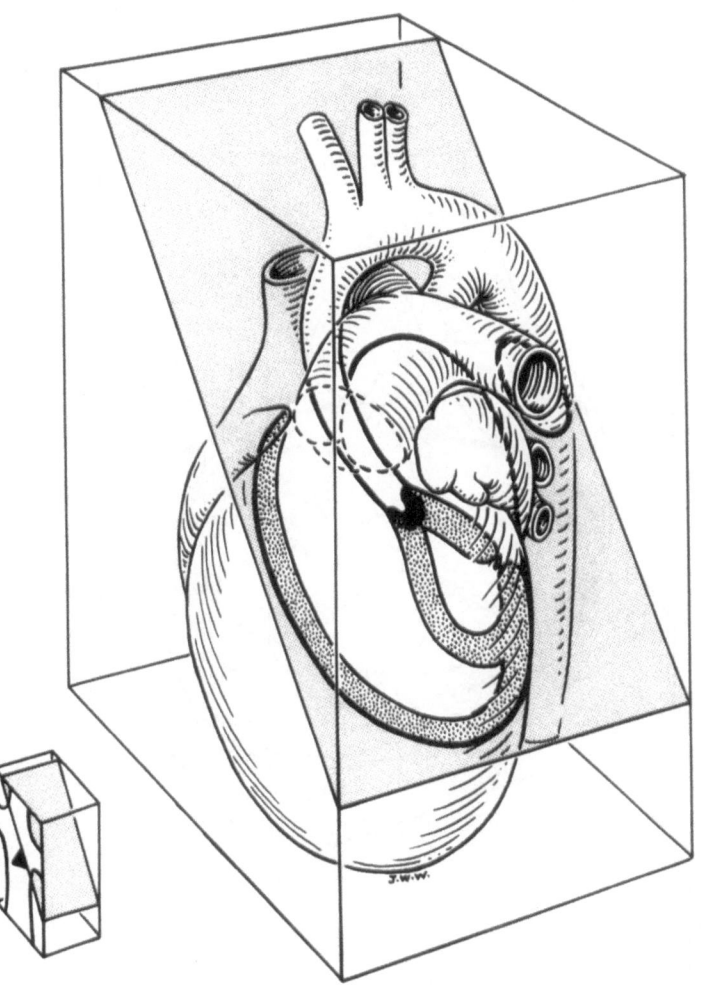

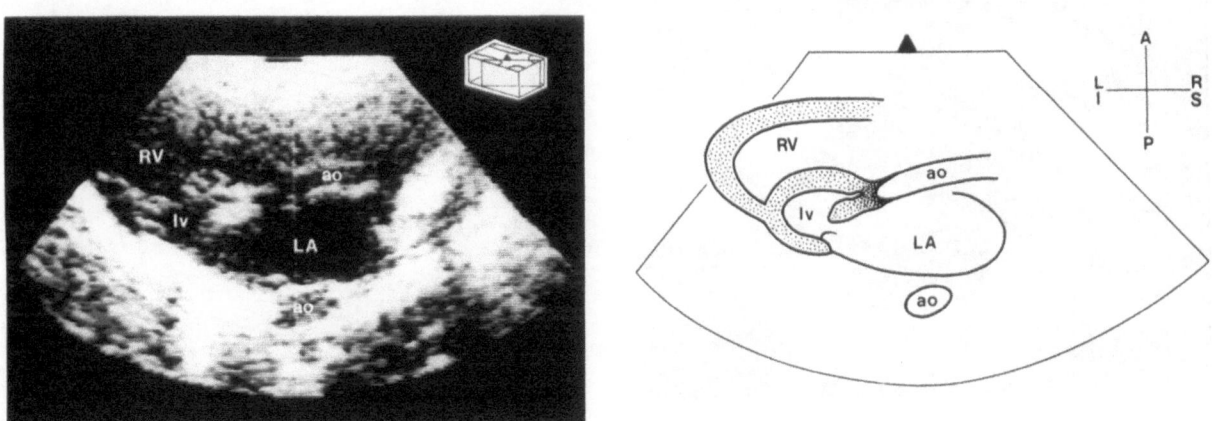

Figure 11.2. Parasternal long axis two-dimensional echocardiogram of the same patient as in Figure 11.1.
 RV = *right ventricle,* lv = *left ventricle,* ao = *aorta,* LA = *left atrium.*

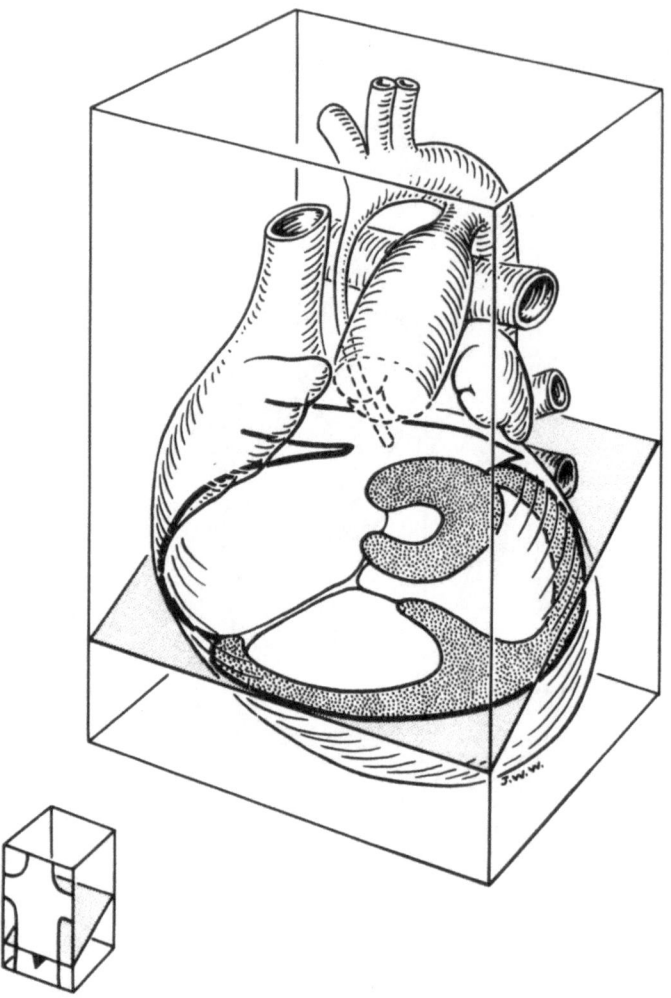

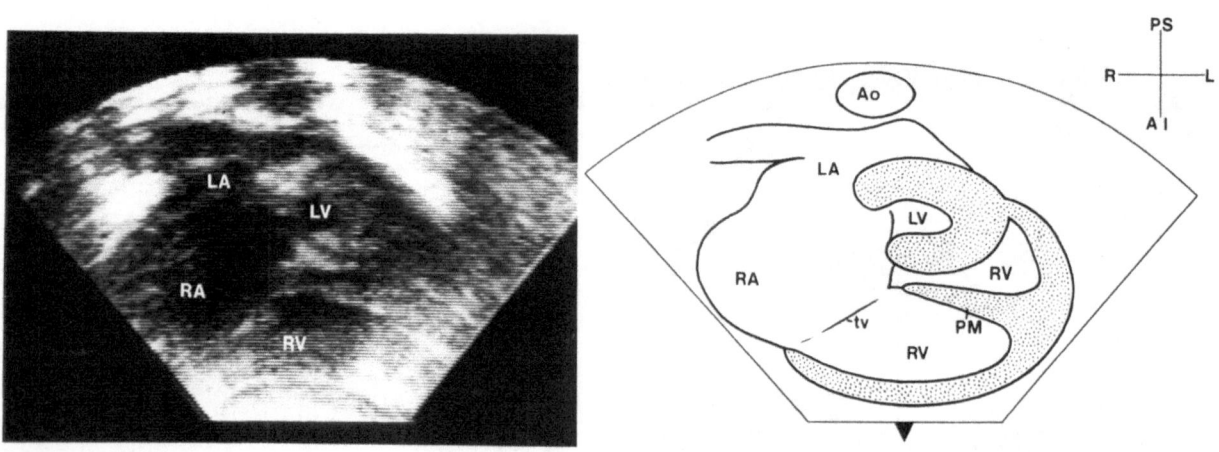

Figure 11.3. Subcostal four chamber two-dimensional echocardiogram of a patient with hypoplastic left heart.

LA = left atrium, LV = left ventricle, RA = right atrium, RV = right ventricle, Ao = aorta, tv = tricuspid valve, PM = papillary muscle.

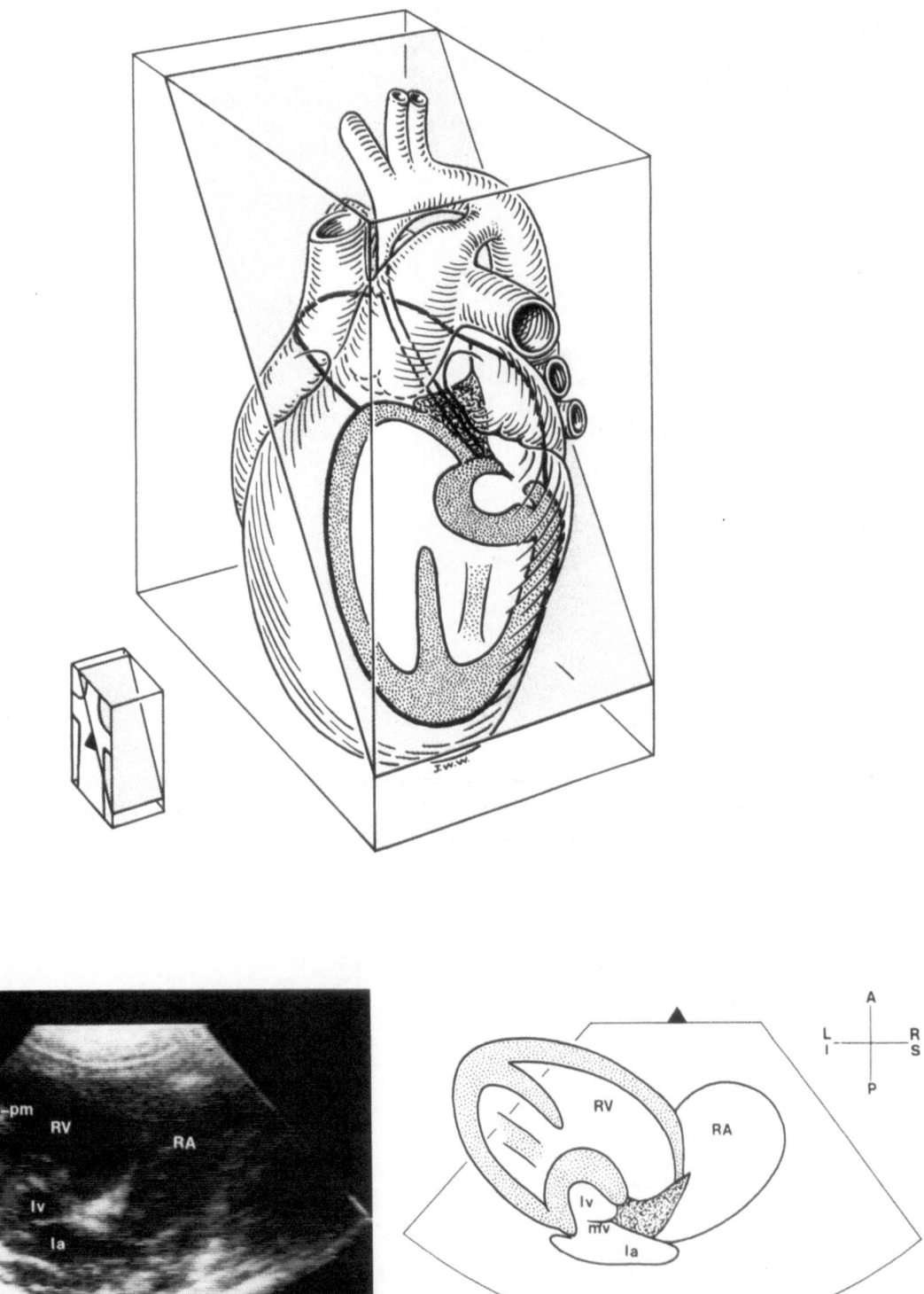

Figure 11.4. Parasternal long axis two-dimensional echocardiogram in the same case as Figure 11.3.

RV = right ventricle, RA = right atrium, lv = left ventricle, la = left atrium, pm = papillary muscle, mv = mitral valve remnant.

126

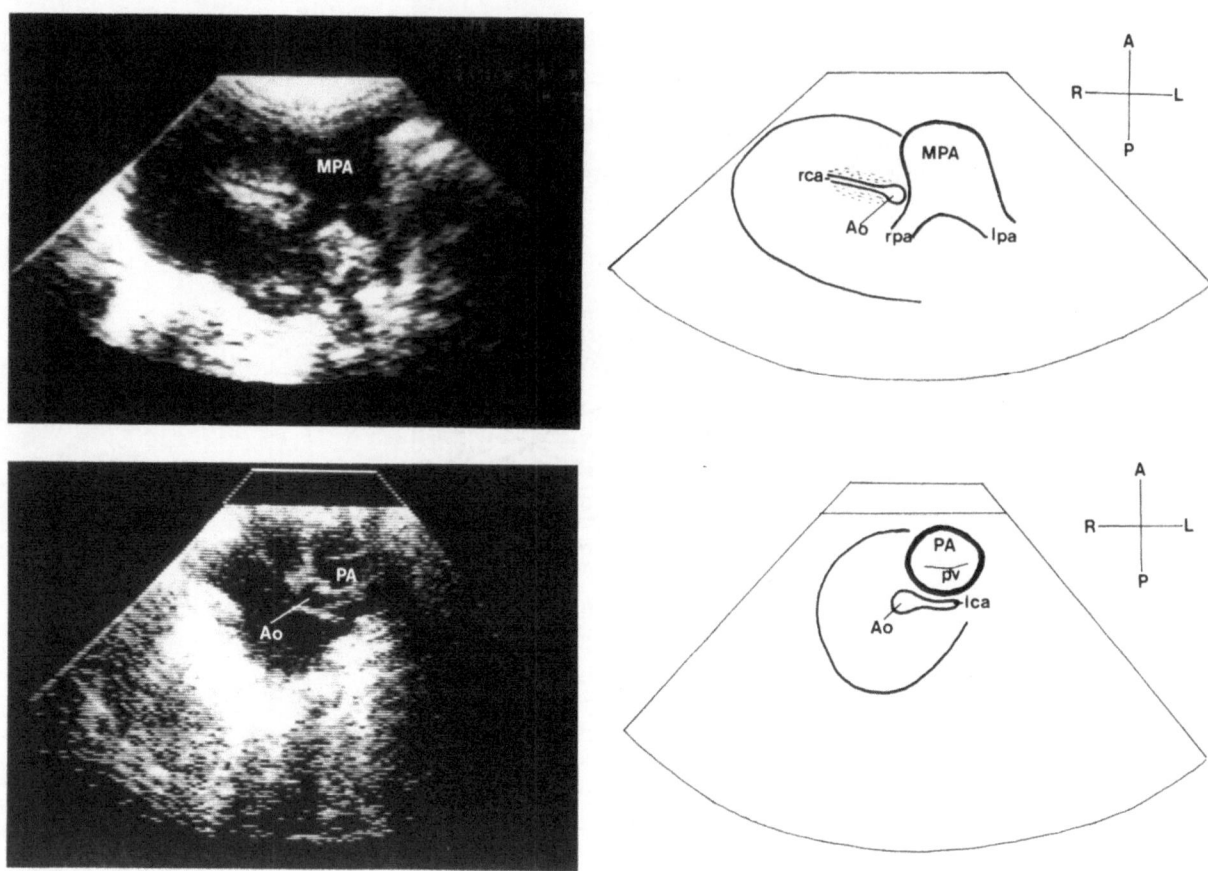

Figure 11.5. Parasternal short axis two-dimensional echocardiograms in infants with hypoplastic left heart syndrome.

PA = pulmonary artery, MPA = main pulmonary artery, lpa = left pulmonary artery, rpa = right pulmonary artery, Ao = aorta, rca = right coronary artery, pv = pulmonary valve, lca = left coronary artery.

12. UNIVENTRICULAR HEART

The term univentricular heart covers a variety of structural cardiac defects which have two anomalies in common. Firstly, the inlet part of the interventricular septum is always missing (1). Secondly, only one chamber has an atrioventricular connection (2), whereby, on basis of the atrioventricular morphology, three distinct types can be defined. The atrioventricular connection may consist of two valves giving exit from two atria to one single ventricle. There may be one atrioventricular valve which connects only one atrium to the main chamber with absence of the contralateral valve. The single atrioventricular communication may also be composed of one common atrioventricular valve in the presence of a common atrium or a primum atrial septal defect. In addition to the main chamber there may be another rudimentary chamber without an atrioventricular connection. This cavity is described as the outlet chamber when it gives exit to one or both great arteries. The main chamber is connected with the outlet chamber through an outlet foramen and is separated from it by the remaining parts of the trabecular and outlet septum. On basis of the morphology of the main chamber univentricular hearts may be defined into right ventricular and left ventricular types. In the former the outlet chamber has a posterior and in the latter an anterior location. The indeterminate type does not have a rudimentary or outlet chamber. Several types of ventriculo-arterial connections exist.

The clinical presentation of a patient with univentricular heart is mainly dependent on the pulmonary perfusion which is determined by the presence or absence of pulmonary obstruction. Without obstruction the volume load of the pulmonary circulation and the heart will be markedly augmented and may give rise to cardiac failure. Obstruction may cause an almost normal or markedly reduced pulmonary blood flow. The extent of the resulting cyanosis depends on the degree of obstruction. Patients with univentricular heart who are severely symptomatic very early in life often have a concomitant lesion such as critical coarctation of the aorta or pulmonary atresia. When the electrocardiogram of an infant shows left ventricular hypertrophy without right ventricular activity a univentricular heart of the left ventricular type, usually with absence of the right sided atrioventricular connection is strongly suggested. Univentricular hearts of the right ventricular type may have electrocardiograms compatible with right ventricular hypertrophy. Univentricular heart is readily diagnosed by two-dimensional echocardiography (3, 4, 5). Multiple views are necessary to appreciate the exact morphology.

In Figure 12.1 a parasternal 'four chamber' view is shown in which a common atrioventricular valve gives exit to both atria. The centrally located atrial septum has ventrally a free edge indicating a primum atrial septal defect. In real-time imaging the two atrioventricular valve leaflets separated during diastole and advanced medially towards each other apposing the ventral edge of the atrial septum during systole.

A similar parasternal 'four chamber' view of a univentricular heart with two atrioventricular orifices is shown in Figure 12.2, whereby the ultrasonic beam struck both valves almost transversely. Therefore, the separate communications between the two atria and the single ventricle are not visualized. The essential feature to be observed here is the presence of the left and the right medial leaflets within the single ventricle without interventricular septum between them. During maximal diastolic opening the medial leaflets were lying in direct apposition. Septal remnants were absent in all

128

other views in this case. The accompanying long axis view shows that the wide anterior aorta and the posterior slender main pulmonary artery arise from the single ventricle in the absence of an outlet chamber.

The subcostal view of a univentricular heart with two atrioventricular valves in Figure 12.3 clearly demonstrates the separate connections of the two atria with the single ventricle. There is no sign of even a remnant of the interventricular septum. Real-time imaging of the atrioventricular valve movements revealed a tunnel shaped narrowing of the left valve as shown in the diastolic frame. The transverse cut through the two atrioventricular orifices also clearly shows the difference in size between the small left and the large right orifice.

A complete echocardiographic analysis of the univentricular heart using the apical and subcostal views is displayed in Figure 12.4. The two atrioventricular valves are shown simultaneously in the apical view. In this case the left orifice is also smaller than the right. Real-time imaging revealed a marked restriction of the movements of the small left atrioventricular valve because of its insertion into only one papillary muscle. The subcostal longitudinal view exposes the main chamber with the posterior main pulmonary artery. Superiorly and to the left a small chamber is visible which is connected to the main chamber through the outlet foramen. The subcostal frontal view discloses the connection between this small chamber and the left-sided anterior aorta, indicating the presence of a subaortic outlet chamber.

Multiple views of univentricular heart with absent right atrioventricular connection are displayed in Figure 12.5. The 'four chamber' view clearly visualizes only three compartments: the right atrium with a venous valve within its cavity and the left atrium which is connected with a single ventricle through a left-sided atrioventricular valve. The posterior relation of the main pulmonary artery and its connection with the main chamber is shown in the subcostal longitudinal view. No further analysis was possible from the subcostal window. The precordial transverse view reveals the left-sided and anterior relationship of the aorta to the main pulmonary artery. By shifting the transducer into the parasternal long axis view an anteriorly located subaortic outflow chamber is visualized.

The outlet chamber is connected through the outlet foramen with the main chamber. The anterior location of the outlet chamber categorized this defect as univentricular heart of the left ventricular type. This type of defect has often been referred to in the past as tricuspid atresia with l-transposition of the great arteries. In cases of tricuspid atresia with a normal relation of the great arteries the rudimentary outlet chamber is continuous with the main pulmonary artery. The communication between the main chamber and the small outlet chamber is usually readily appreciated from the subcostal 'four chamber' and longitudinal views (Figure 12.6).

Univentricular heart with absent right atrioventricular connection is seen in the 'four chamber view' in Figure 12.7. The venous echocontrast injection reveals the obligatory R-L atrial shunt. Such an obligatory R-L atrial shunt is also present in pulmonary atresia with intact interventricular septum. This condition must not be misconstrued as tricuspid atresia with normal relationship of the great arteries. In this defect the pulmonary valve is atretic and there is marked hypoplasia of the right ventricular inflow tract. The tricuspid orifice is small and the chordae and papillary muscles are short. The hypoplastic tricuspid valve may be absent in the normal subcostal four chamber plane because of its superior position compared with the normal, thus, erroneously suggesting absence of the right atrioventricular orifice. In these cases the small tricuspid valve should be searched for in the subcostal longitudinal and frontal and in the parasternal views (Figure 12.8 and 12.9).

References

1. Anderson RH, Becker AE, Wilkinson JL, Gerlis LM: Morphogenesis of univentricular hearts. Br Heart J 38:558 – 572, 1976.
2. Wilkinson JL, Becker AE, Tynan M, Freedom R, Macartney FJ, Shinebourne EA, Quero Gimenez M, Anderson RH, Nomenclature of the univentricular heart. Herz 4:107 – 112, 1979.
3. Sahn DJ, Harder J, Freedom R, Duncan W, Rowe R: Cross-sectional echocardiographic recognition of septal structures in univentricular heart. In: The ventricular septum of the heart, 225 – 233. ACG Wenink et al (eds.). Martinus Nijhoff Publishers, The Hague/Boston/London, 1981.
4. Smallhorn JF, Tommasini G, Macartney FJ: Two-dimen-

sional echocardiographic assessment of common atrioventricular valves in univentricular hearts. Br Heart J 46:30 – 34, 1981.

5. Rigby ML, Anderson RH, Gibson D, Jones ODH, Joseph MC, Shinebourne EA: Two-dimensional echocardiographic categorisation of univentricular heart, ventricular morphology, type, and mode of atrioventricular connection. Br Heart J 46:603 – 612, 1981.

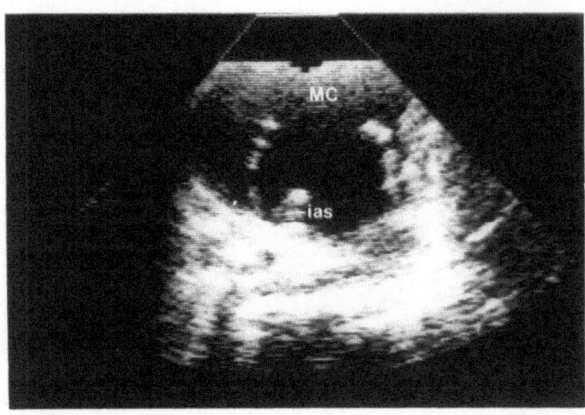
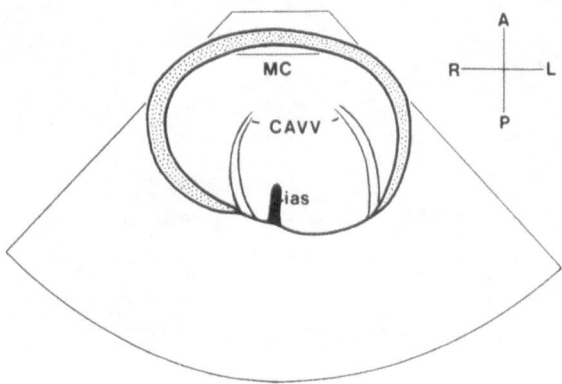

Figure 12.1. Parasternal four chamber two-dimensional echocardiogram of a patient with univentricular heart and a common atrioventricular valve.

MC = main chamber, CAVV = common atrioventricular valve, ias = interatrial septum.

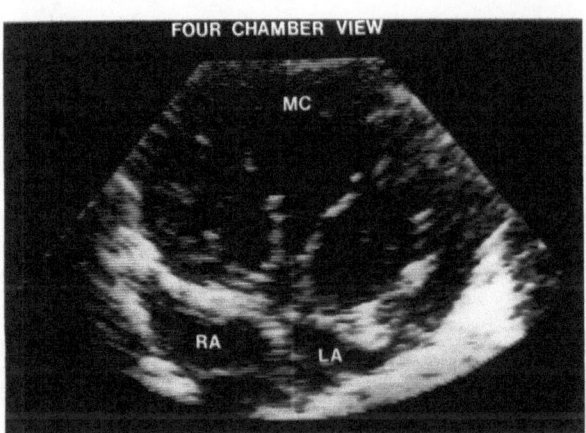
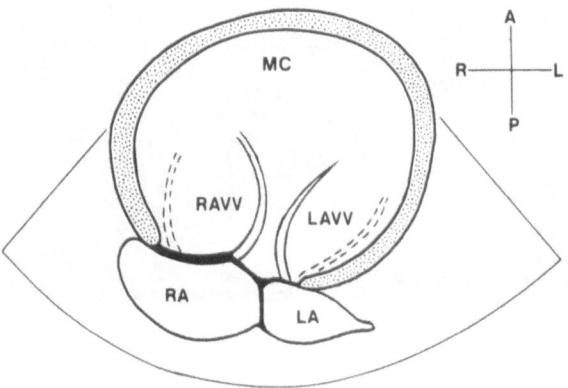
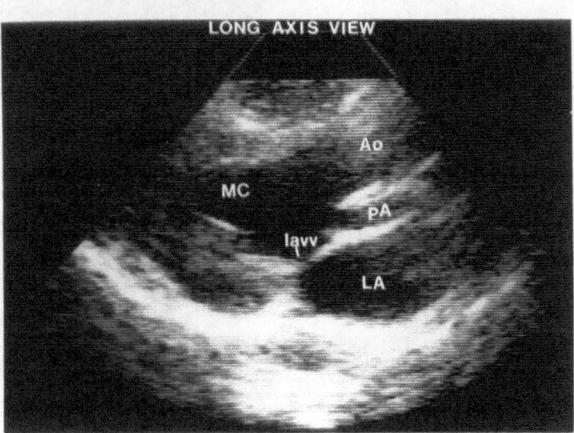

Figure 12.2. Parasternal two-dimensional echocardiograms of a patient with univentricular heart with two atrioventricular valves and without a rudimentary or outflow chamber.

MC = main chamber, RAVV = right atrioventricular valve, LAVV, lavv = left atrioventricular valve, RA = right atrium, LA = left atrium, Ao = aorta, PA = pulmonary artery.

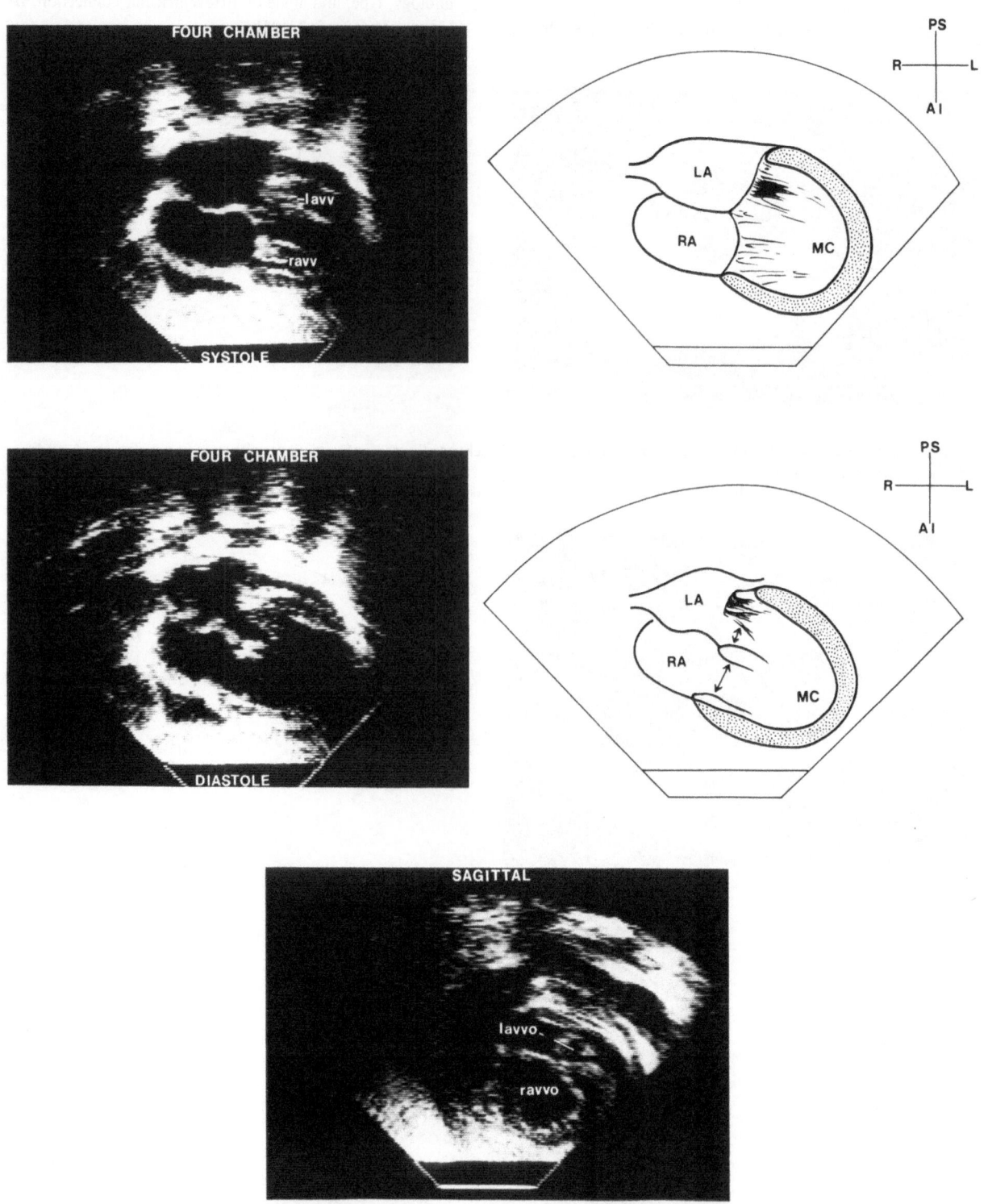

Figure 12.3. Subcostal four chamber view in systole and diastole and subcostal sagittal view in diastole of a patient with univentricular heart and two atrioventricular valves.

LA = left atrium, RA = right atrium, MC = main chamber, lavv = left atrioventricular valve, ravv = right atrioventricular valve, lavo = left atrioventricular orifice, ravo = right atrioventricular orifice.

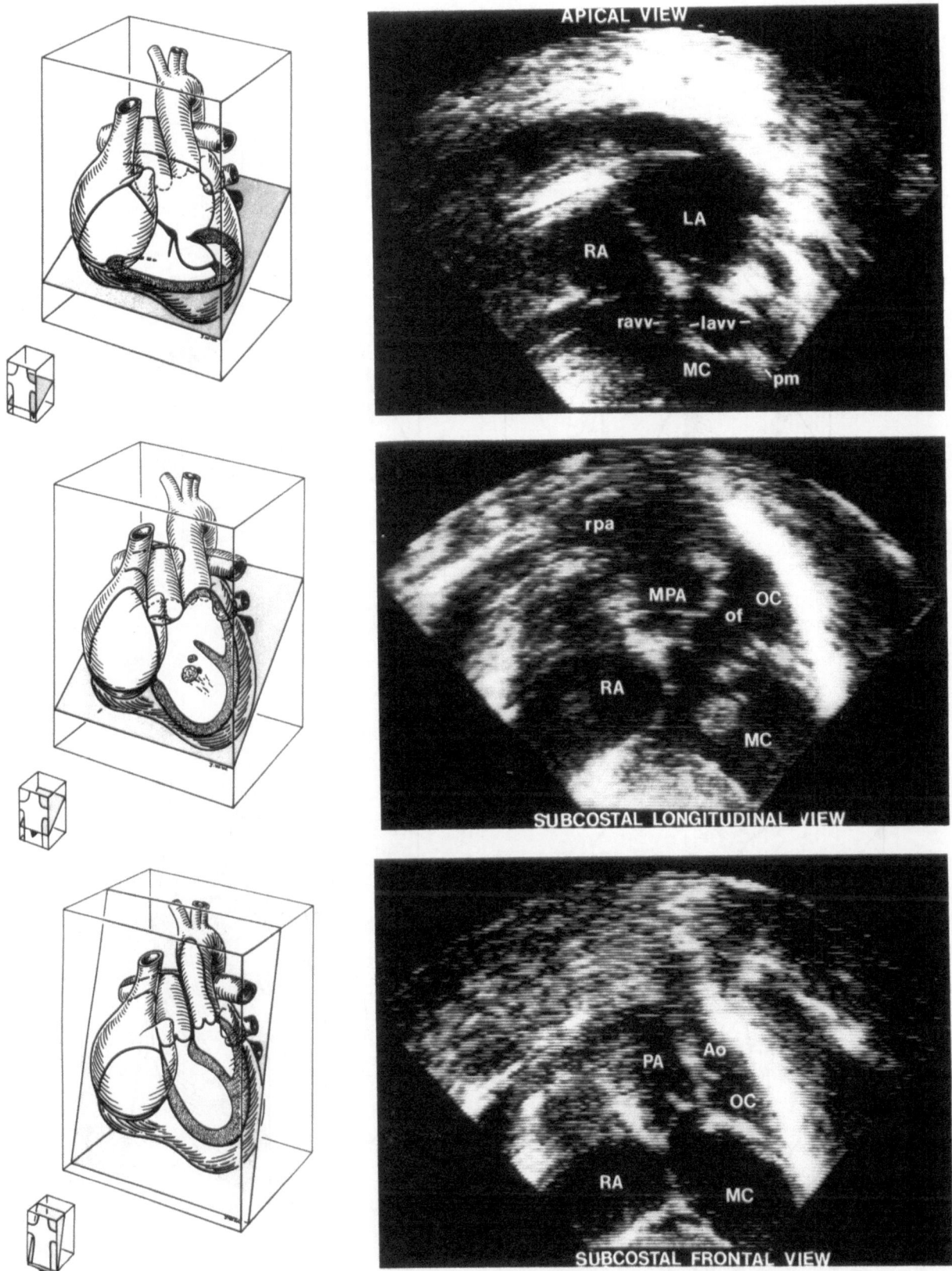

Figure 12.4. Two-dimensional echocardiograms of a patient with univentricular heart, two atrioventricular valves and an anteriorly located subaortic outflow chamber.

RA = right atrium, LA = left atrium, MC = main chamber, ravv = right atrioventricular valve, lavv = left atrioventricular valve, pm = papillary muscle, PA = pulmonary artery, MPA = main pulmonary artery, rpa = right pulmonary artery, OC = outlet chamber, of = outlet foramen, Ao = aorta.

132

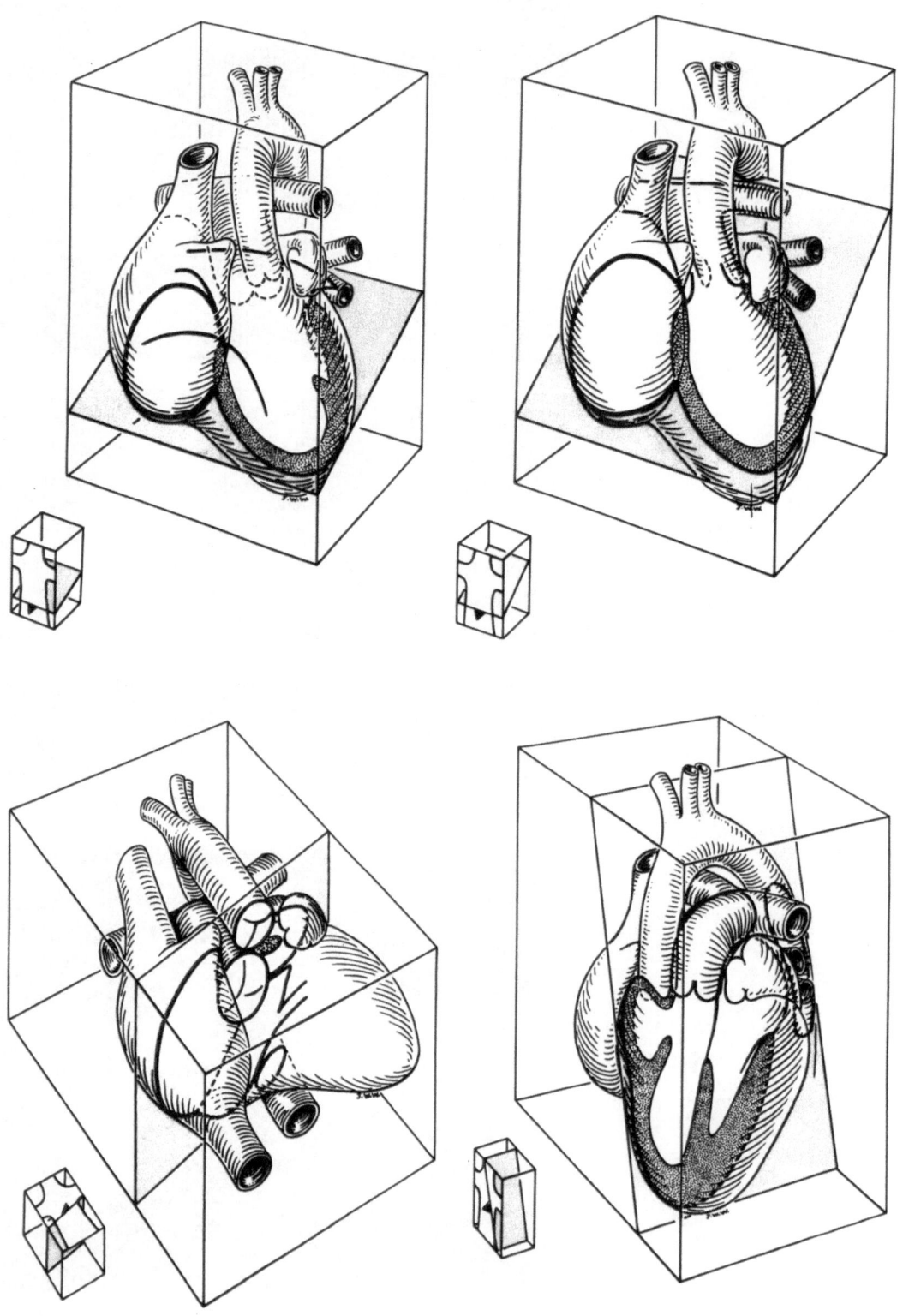

Figure 12.5. For legend see next page.

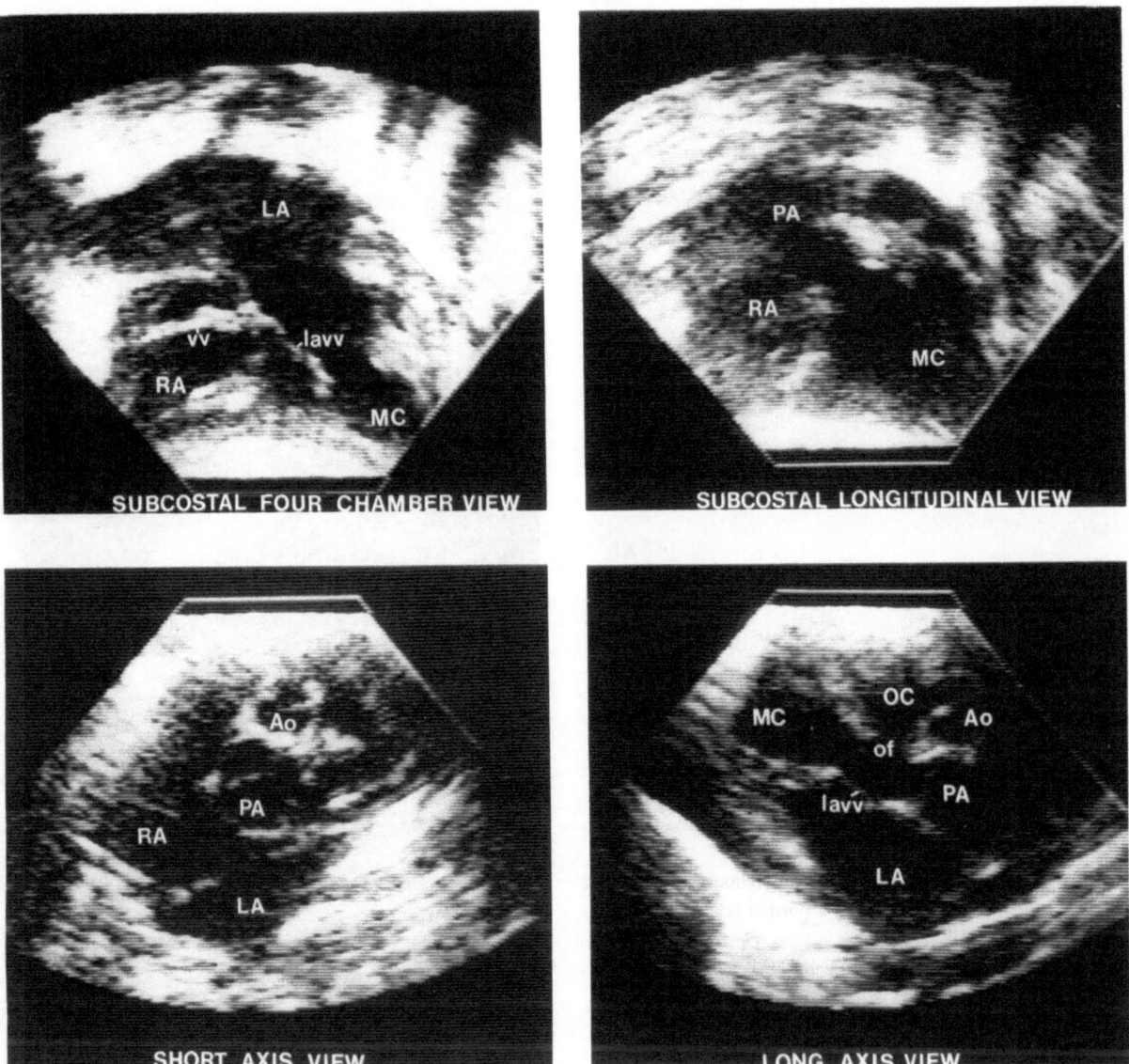

Figure 12.5. Two-dimensional echocardiograms of a patient with tricuspid atresia and l-transposition of the great arteries.

LA = left atrium, RA = right atrium, MC = main chamber, vv = venous valve, lavv = left atrioventricular valve, PA = pulmonary artery, Ao = aorta, OC = outlet chamber, of = outlet foramen.

134

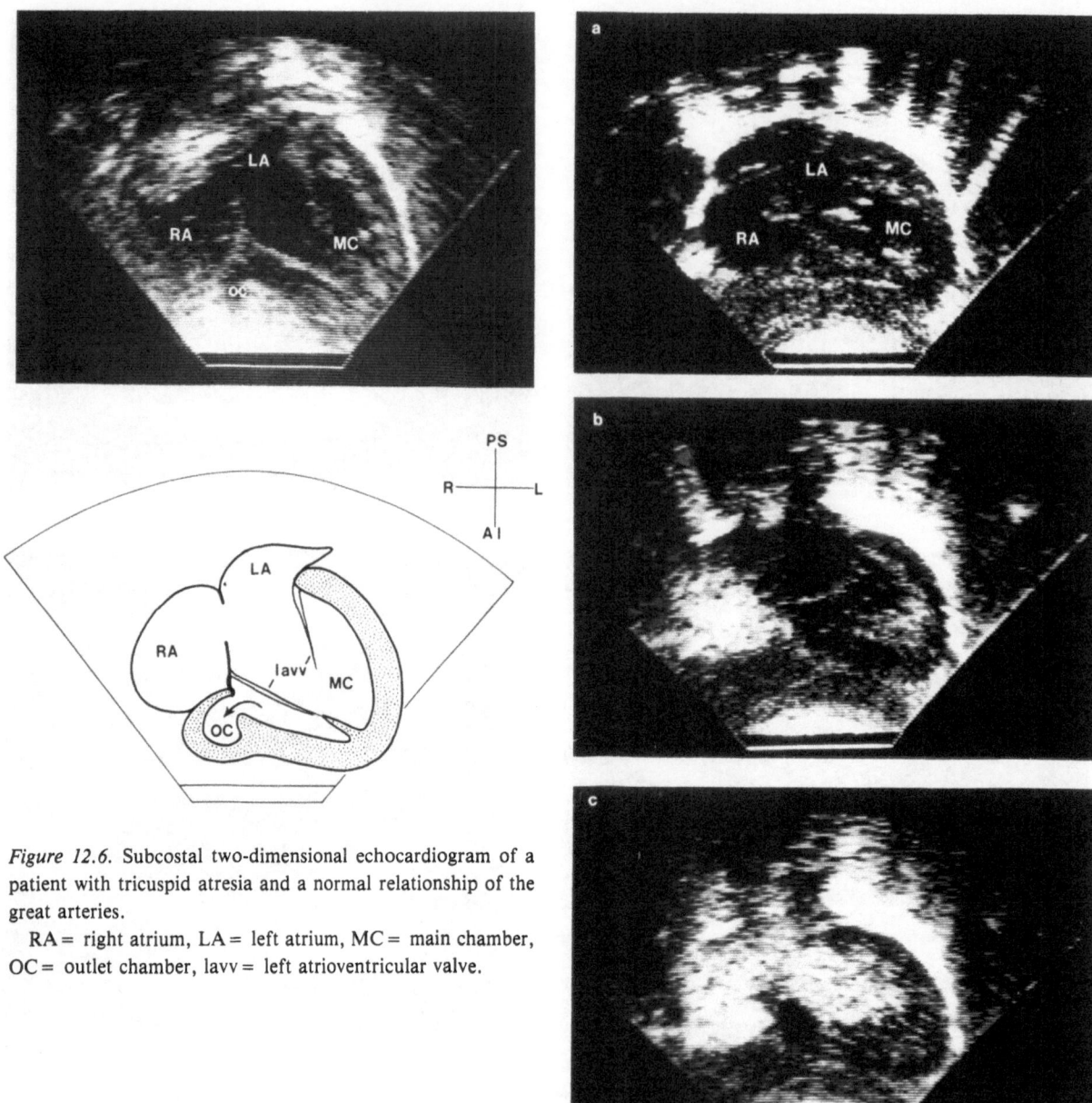

Figure 12.6. Subcostal two-dimensional echocardiogram of a patient with tricuspid atresia and a normal relationship of the great arteries.

RA = right atrium, LA = left atrium, MC = main chamber, OC = outlet chamber, lavv = left atrioventricular valve.

Figure 12.7. Subcostal two-dimensional echocardiograms of a patient with tricuspid atresia before (a) and after (b, c) a venous echocontrast injection. In panel b the contrast has reached the right atrium and in panel c the contrast has passed the atrial septum into the left-sided compartments.

RA = right atrium, LA = left atrium, MC = main chamber.

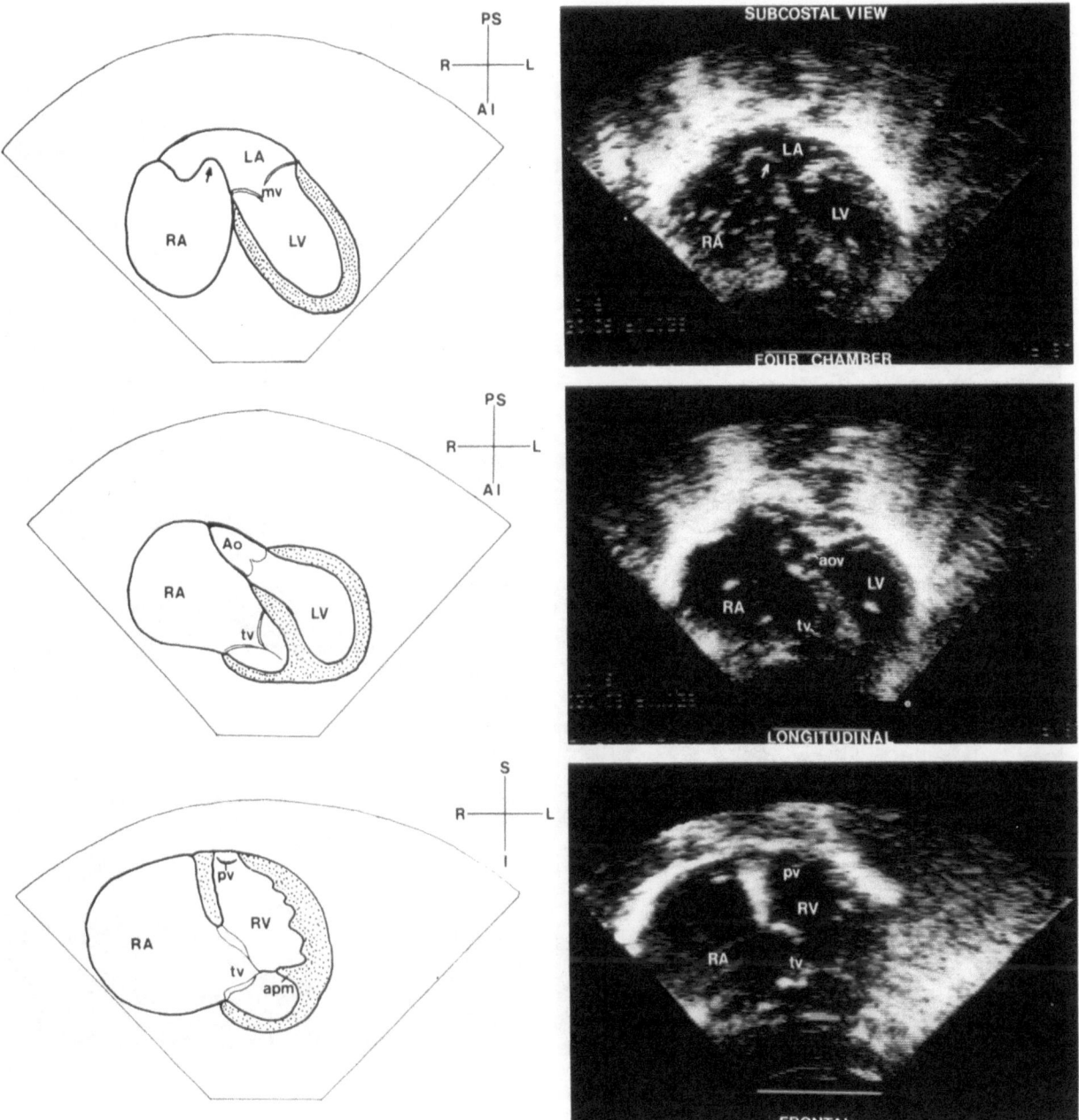

Figure 12.8. Two-dimensional echocardiograms of a patient with pulmonary atresia and intact interventricular septum. The four chamber view does not disclose a tricuspid valve. The central part of the atrial septum forms an aneurysm (arrow) bulging to the left. In the longitudinal view, however, a small tricuspid valve is visible. The right atrium is huge. The frontal view still reveals the hypoplastic tricuspid valve with its insertion with short chordae into a short papillary muscle.

LA = left atrium, RA = right atrium, LV = left ventricle, aov = aortic valve, tv = tricuspid valve, pv = pulmonary valve, RV = right ventricle, apm = anterior papillary muscle.

136

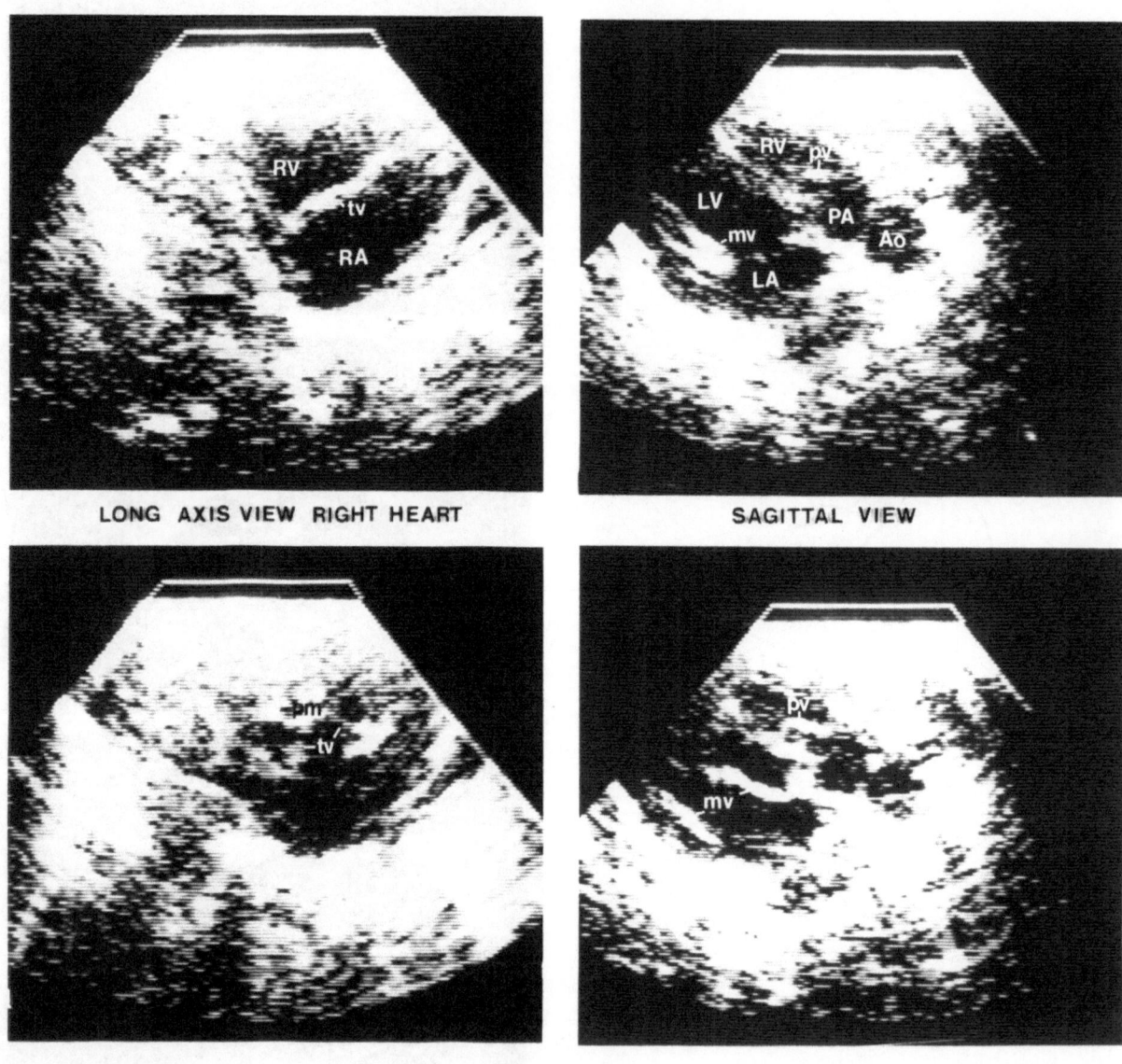

Figure 12.9. Parasternal two-dimensional echocardiogram of a patient with pulmonary atresia and intact interventricular septum. The long axis view of the right heart discloses the hypoplastic tricuspid valve. The diastolic still frame shows clearly the small orifice and the short distance between the tricuspid valve ring and the short papillary muscle. In the sagittal views the normal mitral valve is shown. The pulmonary valve is thickened and does not move during the cardiac cycle.

RV = right ventricle, pv = pulmonary valve, PA = pulmonary artery, Ao = aorta, LV = left ventricle, mv = mitral valve, LA = left atrium.

13. CONGENITALLY CORRECTED TRANSPOSITION
OF THE GREAT ARTERIES

In congenitally corrected transposition of the great arteries, also known as l-transposition, the circulation of blood is normal. The systemic venous blood passes through the right side of the heart, i.e. the right atrium and anatomical left ventricle, to the lungs. The pulmonary venous blood enters the left atrium and flows through the anatomical right ventricle into the aorta. The anomaly can be described as an atrioventricular discordance with ventriculo-arterial discordance. The mitral valve with its two leaflets remains within the anatomical left ventricle and the tricuspid valve with its three leaflets remains part of the anatomical right ventricle.

Usually, these patients are seen by the cardiologist because of additional cardiovascular malformations e.g. ventricular septal defect, pulmonary stenosis, tricuspid incompetence or conduction disturbances such as total atrioventricular block. The diagnosis should be suspected when the electrocardiogram reveals q-waves in the right precordial instead of in the left precordial leads as a result of the reversed activation of the interventricular septum. The upper left border of the cardiac silhouette is abnormally prominent on the chest X-ray because of the left-sided and anterior position of the aorta.

The anatomical left and right ventricles can be identified by two-dimensional echocardiography based on the atrioventricular morphology and attachments, the arrangement of the papillary muscles and the trabecularisation of the ventricular walls (1, 2).

Subcostal two-dimensional echocardiograms of a patient with uncomplicated congenitally corrected transposition of the great arteries are shown in Figure 13.1. The right-sided atrioventricular valve is attached more superiorly to the interventricular septum than the left-sided one which is shown in the four chamber view. This is in contradistinction to the normal heart and identifies the right-sided atrioventricular valve as the mitral valve. The left-sided atrioventricular valve is inserted into a long and centrally located papillary muscle indicating the anterior papillary muscle of the right ventricle. When the transducer was angulated from the four chamber view slightly anteriorly to the longitudinal view the left atrium was replaced by the main pulmonary artery and its bifurcation originating from the right-sided ventricle, thus revealing its posterior location. This view also shows the direct continuity of the right-sided atrioventricular valve with the pulmonary artery which identifies this valve again as the mitral valve. Tilting the ultrasound beam to the frontal plane the aorta is seen anteriorly and to the left of the main pulmonary artery arising from the left-sided ventricle. The wall of this ventricle shows a slightly irregular endocardial surface. Within that ventricle a prominent muscle bundle crossing from the interventricular septum to the left ventricular free wall is visualized. This is the trabecula septomarginalis, an integral part of the right ventricular morphology.

These three subcostal images clearly identify the ventricular morphology and the position of the great arteries. Short axis views of the atrioventricular orifices may provide valuable information in the differentiation of the atrioventricular valves. These transverse views show the rather triangular shape of the tricuspid orifice and the fish-mouth appearance of the bicuspid mitral valve. The sagittal view through the anatomical right ventricle will reveal the discontinuity between the tricuspid orifice and the aorta.

In Figure 13.2 the subcostal four chamber view is shown of a patient with a congenitally corrected transposition of the great arteries, total atrioven-

138

tricular block and severe tricuspid incompetence. The mitral valve is attached to the interventricular septum at the crux of the heart at a higher level than the tricuspid valve. However, the marked distance between these attachments indicates the abnormal low implantation of the tricuspid valve into the interventricular septum. This suggests an Ebstein-like malformation of the tricuspid valve.

The subcostal images in Figure 13.3 depict a 'complicated' ventricular inversion. The four chamber view clearly shows the central insertion of the left atrioventricular valve into the apex of the left-sided ventricle. The right atrioventricular valve is attached to the laterally located papillary muscle group. Therefore, the right and left valves are respectively the mitral and tricuspid valves. The different levels of attachment of the atrioventricular valves onto the interventricular septum is not seen here because the ventricular septal defect extends into the inlet septum. There is also a central atrial septal defect. If the ultrasonic beam is directed anteriorly the pulmonary artery is seen instead of the left atrium. This posterior pulmonary artery is situated on the left side of the trabecular septum and arises from the left-sided anatomical right ventricle. The small outlet septum is just

beneath and to the left of the main pulmonary artery. Hence, the ventricular septal defect may be regarded as a malalignment defect. Pulmonary valve echo's were not seen in the pulmonary orifice. Thus, the echo's seen here were regarded to be subvalvular obstructing muscle or connective tissue. The subcostal frontal view revealed the left-sided and anteriorly located aorta with a normal semilunar valve. Thus, the systematic subcostal echocardiographic analysis disclosed a double outlet of the right ventricle with ventricular inversion, malalignment ventricular septal defect, central atrial septal defect and subpulmonary obstruction.

References

1. Hagler DJ, Tajik AJ, Seward JB, Edwards WD, Mair DD, Ritter DG: Atrioventricular and ventriculoarterial discordance (Corrected transposition of the great arteries). Wide-angle two-dimensional echocardiographic assessment of ventricular morphology. Mayo Clin proc 56:591–600, 1981.
2. Foale R, Stefanini L, Rickards A, Somerville J: Left and right ventricular morphology in complex congenital heart disease defined by two-dimensional echocardiography. Am J Card 49:93–99, 1982.

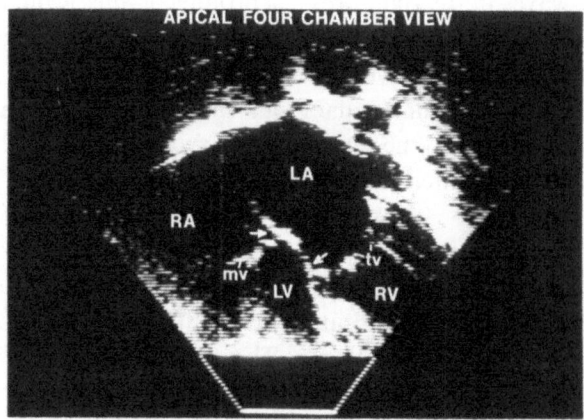

Figure 13.2. Two-dimensional echocardiogram in a patient with congenitally corrected transposition of the great arteries. The arrows in the right and left atrium indicate respectively the site of the septal attachments of mitral and tricuspid valve. The left atrium is enlarged by the apical displacement of the tricuspid valve.

RA = right atrium, LA = left atrium, LV = left ventricle, RV = right ventricle, mv = mitral valve, tv = tricuspid valve.

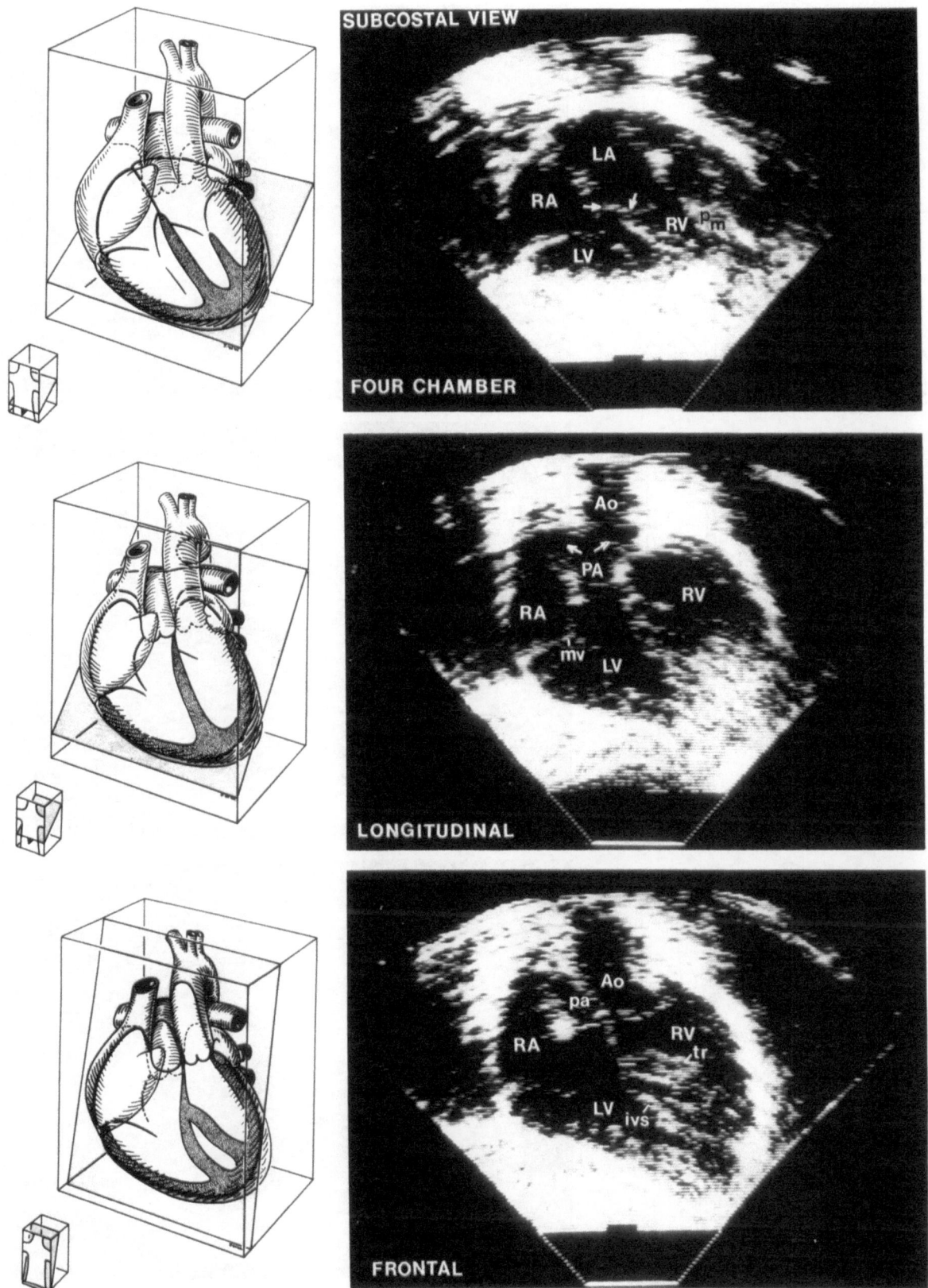

Figure 13.1. Subcostal two-dimensional echocardiograms of a patient with congenitally corrected transposition of the great arteries. In the four chamber view the arrows in the right atrium and in the left atrium indicate respectively the site of the septal attachments of mitral and tricuspid valves. The arrows in the longitudinal view indicate the branches of the pulmonary artery.

RA = right atrium, LA = left atrium, LV = left ventricle, RV = right ventricle, pm = papillary muscle, mv = mitral valve, Ao = aorta, PA, pa = pulmonary artery, ivs = interventricular septum, tr = trabecula septomarginalis.

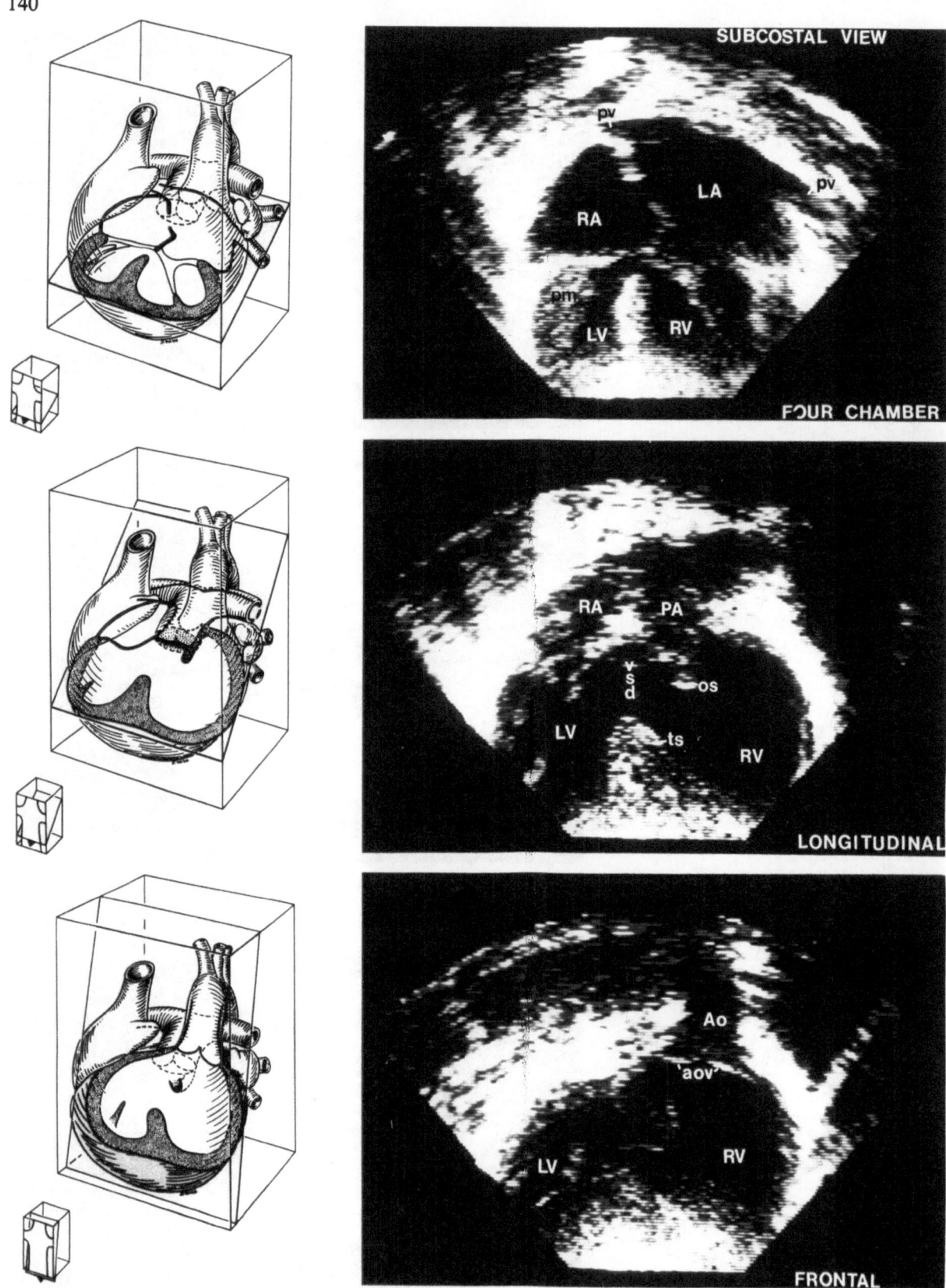

Figure 13.3. Two-dimensional echocardiograms of a patient who was initially diagnosed as univentricular heart. The subcostal views visualize a large ventricular septal defect and a double outlet of the anatomical right ventricle with ventricular inversion (atrioventricular discordance).

RA = right atrium, LA = left atrium, LV = left ventricle, RV = right ventricle, pv = pulmonary vein, pm = papillary muscle, PA = pulmonary artery, vsd = ventricular septal defect, os = outlet septum, ts = trabecular septum, Ao = aorta, aov = aortic valve.

14. CRISS-CROSS HEART

The term criss-cross heart denotes an uncommon malformation whereby the pulmonary and systemic bloodflows cross each other at atrioventricular level (1). In the case of atrioventricular concordance the right ventricle is situated superiorly to the left ventricle with a horizontally positioned interventricular septum. Blood from the right atrium empties into the right ventricle in a right-inferior to left-superior direction. The atrioventricular connection on the left side, through which the blood stream passes in a posterior to anterior direction, lies inferior to that of the right side.

In cases with atrioventricular discordance the criss-cross atrioventricular relationship is caused by a 'normal' spatial relationship of the two ventricles. The posteriorly located left atrium is connected with the anteriorly located right ventricle and inferior to this connection the right atrium is horizontally linked with the left ventricle from the right to the left side. The ventriculo-arterial connections may vary. Frequently occurring associated lesions are pulmonary stenosis, hypoplastic tricuspid valve and ventricular septal defect.

Figure 14.1 and Figure 14.2 show a subcostal two-dimensional echocardiographic analysis of a newborn child with discrete cyanosis, tachypnoea and cardiomegaly with increased pulmonary vascular markings on the chest X-ray. The electrocardiogram revealed right atrial dilatation and biventricular hypertrophy. The subcostal analysis showed the criss-cross atrioventricular relationship.

The four chamber view (Figure 14.1) does not reveal the tricuspid valve and the right ventricle in the correct position. The bulging of the interatrial septum to the left suggests a right-sided obstructive lesion. Tricuspid atresia is likely to be present. The left atrium is connected to a left and inferiorly located ventricle through an atrioventricular valve inserted into two discrete chordal structures, which can be appreciated in a slightly inferiorly located cross-section (four chamber view in Figure 14.2). These structures protrude into the ventricle and diverge towards the apex suggesting two separate papillary muscles attached to the inferior wall of the ventricle. The image of one centrally and anteriorly oriented papillary muscle, as is normally seen in right ventricular morphology, is clearly missing. Therefore, the ventricle and the atrioventricular valve can be defined as the morphological left ventricle with the mitral valve. Superiorly and to the left of this ventricle a thick-walled small cavity of undefined origin is clearly visible, provisionally labeled as the right ventricle.

By tilting the ultrasonic beam anteriorly to obtain the subcostal longitudinal view, the posteriorly located pulmonary artery, identified by its bifurcation, is visualized. In this view the pulmonary artery originates mainly from the morphological left ventricle. The mitral valve shows here a direct continuity with the right wall of the pulmonary artery, positively identifying this valve. In the left subpulmonary region an obvious communication exists between the left ventricle and the superiorly located small cavity that was provisionally denoted as the right ventricle in the four chamber view.

Further information regarding the cardiac pathology is provided by the subcostal frontal view. It is important to note that a second hypoplastic atrioventricular valve, i.e. the tricuspid valve, is situated in an abnormal superior position just anterior to the pulmonary valve. Via this valve the large right atrium is connected with the presumptive right ventricle, indicating that this chamber actually is the morphological right ventricle. The lateral wall has an irregular surface corresponding with right ventricular trabeculations. Other frontal views (not exhibited here) showed

142

septal insertions of the tricuspid valve. The abnormally positioned small right ventricle gives rise to an anteriorly and to the left located aorta. Another observation is the almost horizontal position of the interventricular septum in the frontal view.

The criss-cross atrioventricular relationship in the case described is evident. The right atrium is anteriorly connected with a small leftsided and superiorly located right ventricle, while the connection between left atrium and left ventricle lies inferiorly directed from posterior-superior to anterior-inferior. Therefore, the final two-dimensional echocardiographic diagnosis is atrioventricular concordance, ventriculo-arterial discordance, ventricular septal defect, hypoplasia of the right ventricle and the tricuspid orifice and a criss-cross atrioventricular relationship.

This unusual case is another example that shows how failure to visualize the tricuspid valve in the normal four chamber plane does not prove the absence of that valve. The hypoplastic tricuspid valve in cases with pulmonary atresia with intact ventricular septum can also have an abnormal superior position (chaper 12).

References

1. Anderson RH, Shinebourne EA, Gerlis LM: Criss-cross atrioventricular relationships producing paradoxical atrioventricular concordance or discordance. Circulation 50: 176 – 180, 1974.

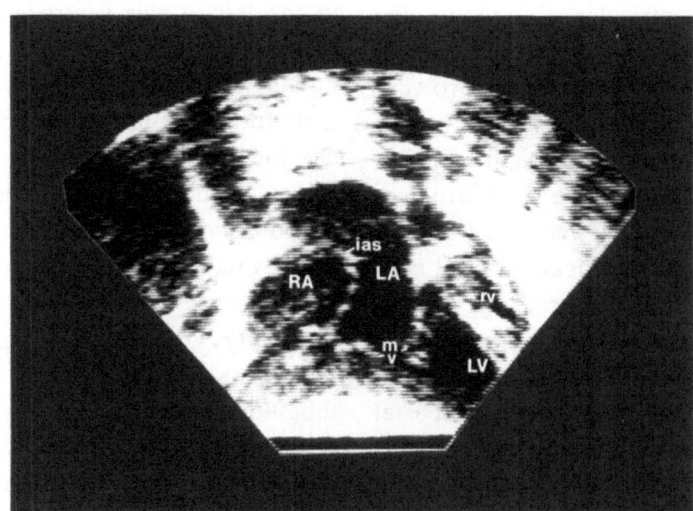

Figure 14.1. Subcostal four chamber two-dimensional echocardiogram of a patient with a criss-cross heart. The interatrial septum bulges as a whole towards the left. The tricuspid valve is absent in this view.

RA = right atrium, ias = interatrial septum, LA = left atrium, mv = mitral valve, LV = left ventricle, rv = right ventricle.

143

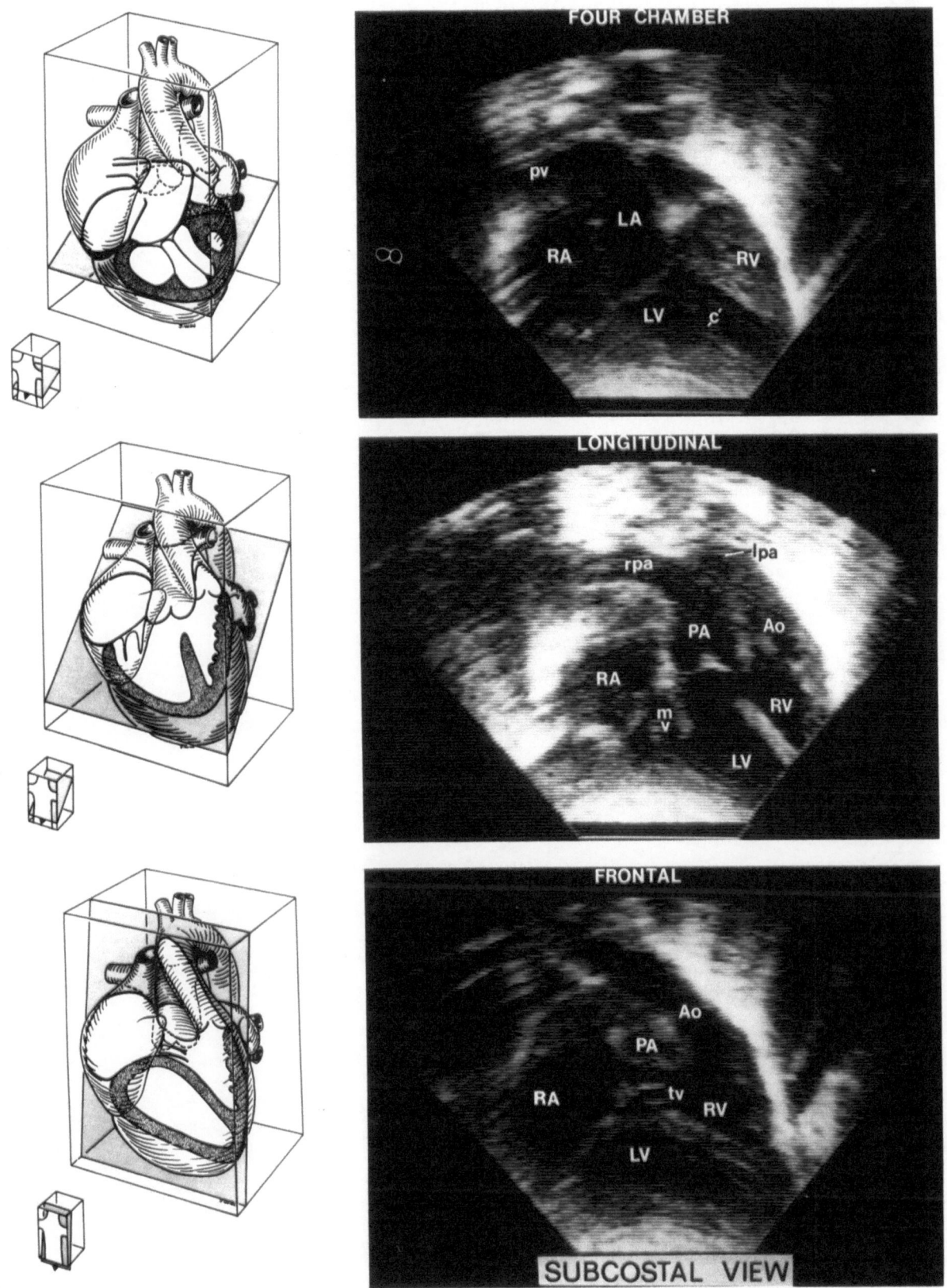

Figure 14.2. Subcostal two-dimensional echocardiograms of the same patient as in Figure 14.1. For further explanation see text.
pv = pulmonary vein, RA = right atrium, LA = left atrium, LV = left ventricle, RV = right ventricle, c = chordae, rpa = right pulmonary artery, lpa = left pulmonary artery, PA = pulmonary artery, Ao = aorta, mv = mitral valve, tv = tricuspid valve.